SAND TRAINING FOR SPORTS

By

Jason Shea M.S, PICP IV

"It isn't the mountain ahead that wears you out; it's the grain of sand in your shoe"

-Rodan of Alexandria

Special thank you Wen, Ayden, and Bryn for all your patience, support, and understanding with the long hours away from home to make this book project happen. Thank you Mom and Dad for your constant inspiration. Thank you to the wonderful staff and community at APECS and CrossFit Tri-Valley for continuously keeping me on my toes and inspiring me to be both a better person and professional. Thank you to all my great friends in the health and wellness industry. Learning from you and being around you as both friend and professional is like carrying a flame that lights the way to continuous improvement. And lastly, I would like to thank Charles Poliquin for opening my eyes to an entirely different level of all things health, wellness, and strength and conditioning. To anybody else I may have missed, I thank you!

Table of Contents

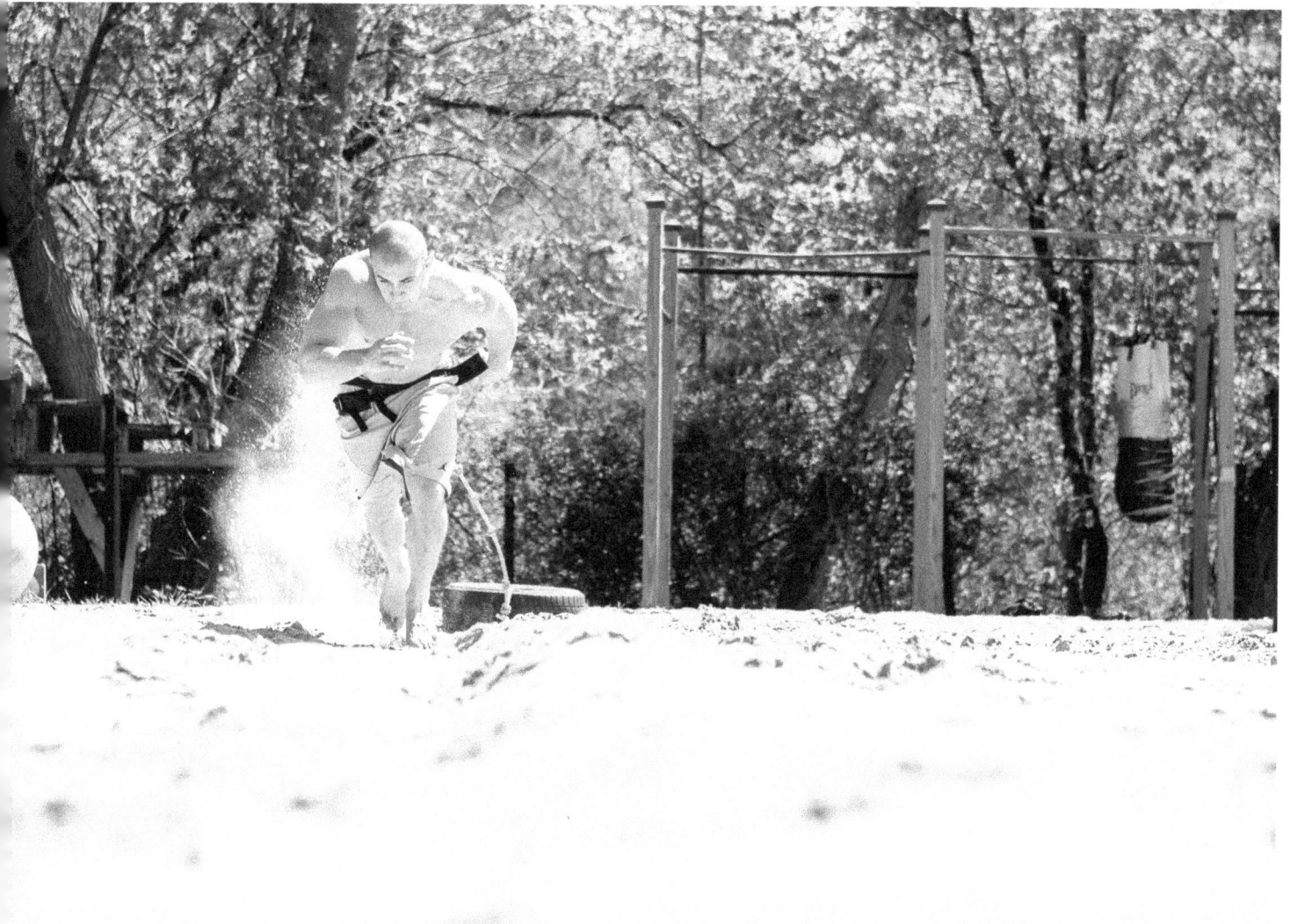

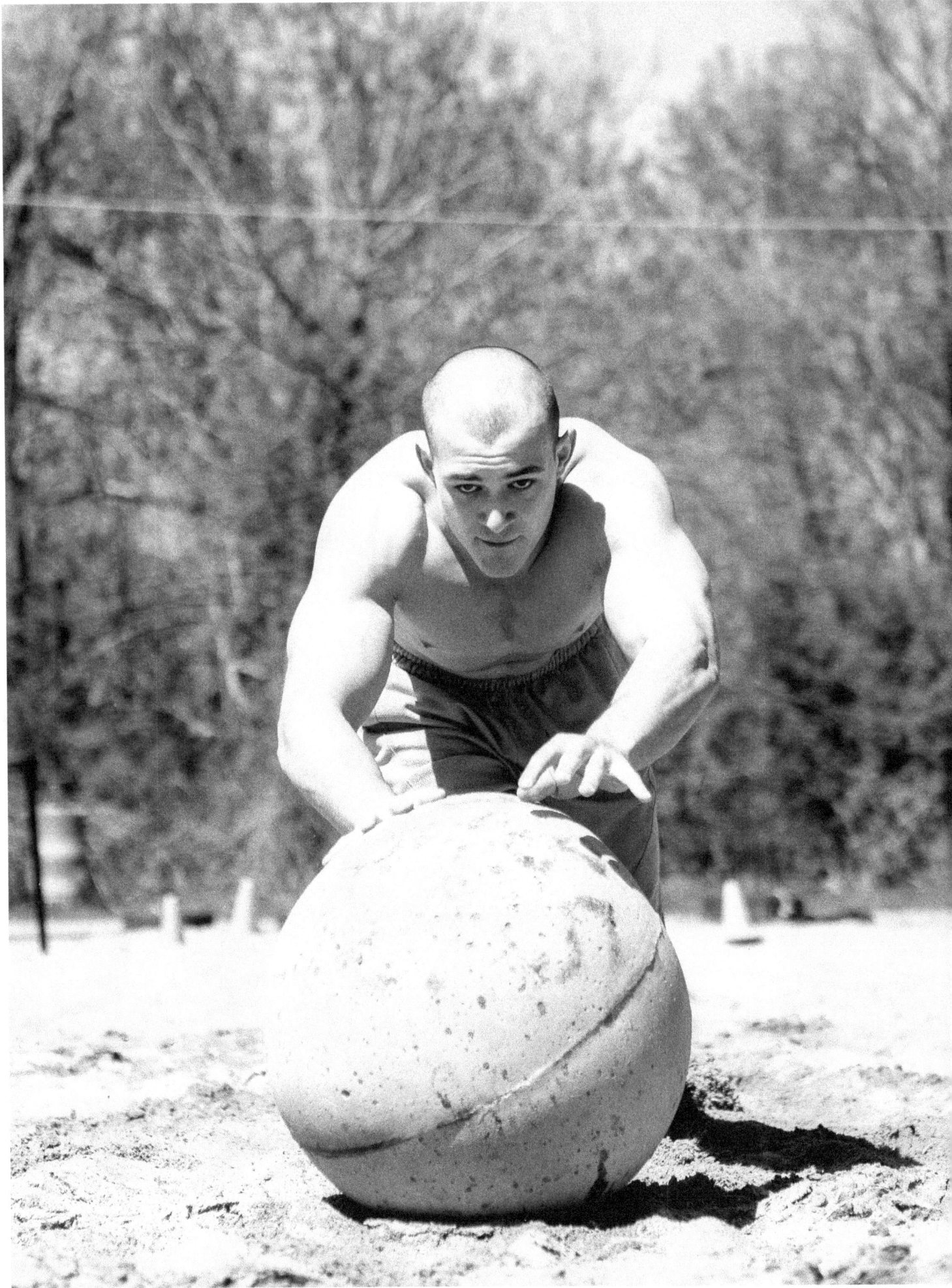

Chapter I

Benefits of Training

in the Sand

Over the years athletes and coaches have continuously looked for newer and more effective training methodologies to gain a competitive edge on the field. From functional training methods utilizing strongman equipment to power enhancement and speed, agility, and quickness drills,

The focus of the majority of these programs is quite simple: to enhance athletic performance and minimize risk of injury. When we think of enhancing athletic performance with regards to the training itself, we think of a variety of factors including:

Training Factors

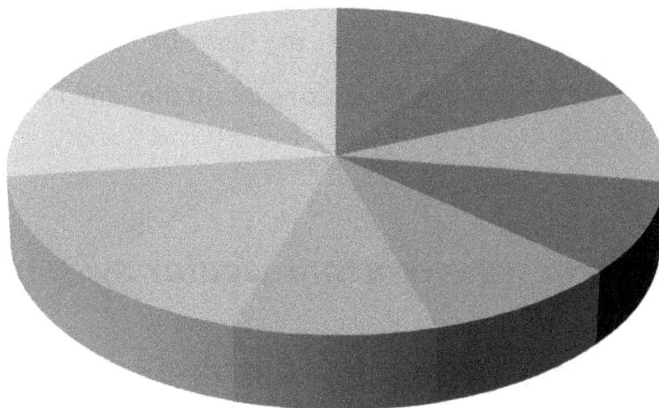

- Movement Quality
- Decrease Injury Risk
- Improve Structural Balance
- Increase "Horsepower"
- Improve Body Composition
- Increase Functional Strength
- Improve Flexibility
- Increase Lean Muscle Mass
- Increase Speed, Agility, and Quickness
- Improve Sport Specific Condition
- Enhance Mental Toughness

General and specific training protocols are used to both enhance strong points and address those factors that need improvement. Olympic weight lifting and plyometric exercises are often used for increasing power. Conventional strength training methods are used to increase horsepower through neuromuscular adaptations and improvements in muscle mass, hormonal profile, and body composition. Structural balance training methods are a great tool for correcting muscular imbalances, rehabilitating current injuries, and preventing future injuries from occurring. Speed, agility, and quickness drills can be used to improve these on-field markers of athletic qualities. Modified strongman modalities are use to enhance functional strength, and therefore bridge the gap between weight room strength and on-field functionality.

Rest interval and intensity dependent, many of the aforementioned training methods can be used for metabolic conditioning purposes, while nearly all of them can be used to build mental toughness and the associated character that comes along with hard work.

One simple, but oft-overlooked element of training that can have a profound impact on intensity and positive athletic improvement is that of training on decreased surface stability, or more specifically training in the sand. The simplest way to describe the significant benefits of working out in the sand is:

According to a 2004 study from *Medicine and Science in Sports and Exercise* the average caloric expenditure for men and women walking or running 1600 meters on a hard surface is: [19]
- **Walking:** Men - 88cal; Women - 74cal
- **Running:** Men - 124cal; Women 105cal

1600 meters on sand would have burned:
- **Walking:** Men – 237.6 cal; Women 199.8 cal
- **Running:** Men – 198 cal; Women 168 cal

Training in the sand forces the neuromuscular system to work harder, therefore garnering better results!

It is no wonder why so many pro athletes and college teams have augmented their weight room and filed workouts with sand training. Take for instance a 2013 comparison study that looked at the pre and post training agility performance of athletes training in the sand versus those training on a hard surface. To test agility the athletes performed the T drill and the 505 drill, both for time. Each group performed the same training 3X per week for 10

Just a few of the College Football Teams that have sandpits:
- Michigan
- Oregon
- Auburn
- Ohio State
- Washington State
- Miami
- Penn State
- Georgia Southern

weeks, with the sand group performing on the sand and the other group on hard surfaces (16). The workout breakdown is below:

Warm Up: General activity on the surface for 15 minutes
Main Part of the Workout: 15min speed/jumping, 45 min technical skill
Cool Down: 15min cool down/stretching

After 10 weeks of training, the results of the T Test hard surface evaluation were:

Group	Pre-Training Hard Surface Testing	5th Week Hard Surface Testing	10th Week Hard Surface Testing	Improvement
Sand Training Group	15.3s	14.4s	13.2s	**2.1s** (**13.8% increase** on hard surface testing!)
Hard Surface Training Group	15.1s	14.7s	14.4s	**.7s**(*only a 4.9% increase on hard surface testing*)

Gortsila E, Apostolos T, Nesic G, Maridaki M. **Effect of training surface on agility and passing skills of prepubescent female volleyball players.** *Sports Medicine and Doping Studies.* 3(2); Pp. 1-5. 2013.

And the results for the 505 agility evaluation on the hard surface were:

Group	Pre-Training Hard Surface Testing	5th Week Hard Surface Testing	10th Week Hard Surface Testing	Improvement
Sand Training Group	3.45s	3.25s	2.98s	**.47s** (**13.8% increase** on hard surface testing!)
Hard Surface Training Group	3.34	3.25	3.18	**.16s**(*only a 4.7% increase on hard surface testing*)

Gortsila E, Apostolos T, Nesic G, Maridaki M. **Effect of training surface on agility and passing skills of prepubescent female volleyball players.** *Sports Medicine and Doping Studies.* 3(2); Pp. 1-5. 2013.

These results show that after 10 weeks of training, the athletes who were training in the sand-only had significantly greater results in hard surface agility testing than did those athletes who were actually training on the hard surfaces (16).

Even though the workout intensities were similar, the researchers concluded that not only were the sand workouts more metabolically demanding, but the proprioceptive demand was also significantly greater as well. The researchers stated "*a non-solid ground, like sand, may evoke changes in the neuromuscular junctions. An unstable surface may lead to repeated losses of balance,*

> The surface stiffness of sand is roughly 3-4 times less than the surface stiffness of grass greater on grass.

which in turn and in order to avoid falling may promote neuromuscular communication and therefor improve balance (16)".

In a 1982 *Sports Illustrated* article, former football legend Walter Payton, expressed similar thoughts, in which he believed that the constant adjustments required for successful sprinting and cutting in the sand were major training contributors to his world-class agility, acceleration, and low rate of injury (42).

By constantly having to adjust posture to the changing surface, sand training not only improves agility, but is also aids in injury prevention due to the increased demand on the stabilizer muscles throughout the kinetic chain. For example, the muscles that stabilize our major shock absorbers, the ankles, are heavily recruited during sand training. The instability of the sand allows for a greater range of motion in all biomechanical actions of the ankle. This increased training load and demand can provide stimulus enough to increases in strength in the musculature about this joint.

A 2006 *LA Times* article on sand training at Manhattan Beach Dune Park discusses the countless professional and Olympic athletes who train on the dune for their off-season and pre-season workouts. Year after year, from basketball MVPs to baseball and hockey stars to football defensive players of the year, these athletes set the example of how beneficial (*and difficult*) sand training can be (12).

According to a 1991 *National Strength and Conditioning Association* article, sand training can lead to an *"increase in proprioception and sensory integration of the lower extremities. Such an increase is a direct product of requiring the ankles to function through their full complement of kinesiological ranges. As opposed to running on artificial turf or regular grass where the ankle is exposed to less variation and therefore fewer proprioceptive adjustments, running in sand requires the ankle's proprioceptors to make constant adjustments with each stride in order to preserve balance as well as running synchronization (33)."*

Every June there is an event off the West Coast of Denmark called the North Sea Beach Marathon. It is 26 miles in heavy and soft sand. The 2013 winner finished in 3:03:02.

The same increase in sensory integration and neuromuscular demand can be said for strengthening about the knee and hip joints. The multidirectional nature of stabilizing on the sand leads increased demands on the musculature about these joints. This in turn can increase the overall stability and integrity of the lower extremities. It is for these reasons that many Orthopedic Doctors and Physical Therapists have recommend their clients toward training in the sand during the later stages of physical therapy.

Another oft-overlooked injury-preventive benefit of sand training is the increased demand of the core and low back musculature. The uneven and unstable surface requires constant adjustments in the ankles, knees, and hips, which in turn leads to small perturbations in the torso. To adjust for these small movements and keep the athlete upright, there is an increased demand on the core and low back musculature in order to stay upright.

The Manhattan Beach Sand Dune Park, otherwise known as "The Dune" has been a select training spot of countless professional and college athletes over the years. The attraction: a 100-foot climb (or sprint) in soft sand up a 45 degree incline.

Accelerating and sprinting in the sand can also aid in correcting structural imbalances between the quadriceps and hamstring musculature. When athletes sprint in the sand there is an increased demand on the hamstring musculature, particularly as extensors of the hips. As sand is a very forgiving surface, an athlete is forced exaggerate hip extension and plantar flexion due to the sliding and sinking of the foot into the sand during the drive phase of sprinting. According to the aforementioned 1991 article from *The National Strength and Conditioning Association Journal* "sprinting in sand exaggerates the various stride components (33)." The authors drew parallels to spinning tires in the mud with regards to the foot sink and slide, and resultant increase in hamstring demand (*more on this later*).

Not only does SAQ training in the sand decrease your risk of injury and make you more agile on turf, grass, and hard courts, but it has also been shown to have a significantly greater caloric expenditure and mechanical work demand. In essence, it provides a much better "*BANG FOR YOUR BUCK*".

Soccer stars and teams from around the globe have been known to hone their skills and train on the sand. Several Soccer Academies in Brazil utilize sand training for their athletes including:
- Zico Soccer Academy
- De Lima Soccer Enterprises Camps
- Oscar Inn Soccer Academy

A 2013 study looked at biomechanics and energy expenditure of soccer players who performed short sprint and shuttle runs on turf, grass, and sand. The researchers found a decrease in the elastic elements involved in sprinting and deceleration mechanics. This increased the mechanical work demand on the subject's neuromuscular systems, leading to a higher energy cost of training. The energy expenditure was estimated to be roughly 30% greater for those training in the sand versus those training on the harder surface (15).

In carrying the theme of energy expenditure on sand versus hard surfaces, in 1998 a Belgian research team set out to determine the differences in human locomotion on sand versus hard surface. Amazingly they found that running on sand was over one and a half times more demanding than running on hard surfaces. In other words running on sand requires more than 1.5 times more energy than running on harder surfaces (27).

The same research team also found that the simple task of walking on sand required nearly two and half times more energy than did walking on hard surfaces (27). In essence, athletes who train in the sand are not only achieving better results in agility, but they are also burning considerably more calories!

> According to a 2005 article from *National Geographic News*, if a person falls into quicksand they will not sink all the way down. Humans are not dense enough. The density of quicksand is about 2 grams per ml, while humans are roughly 1gram per ml. Interestingly, if you do fall in, the amount of force needed to pull your foot out is similar to the forces it would require to lift a small car. This eliminates somebody pulling you out. Rather the researchers suggest wiggling your legs to free yourself (2).

Another measure of workload and workout intensity is Heart Rate. A research team out of Australia measured not only heart rate, but also blood lactate levels of competitive athletes performing 20-meter sprints on grass and sand for an eight week training block. The researchers also tested to see if higher training intensities led to a breakdown in next day performance of the same sprints.

The researchers found heart rate to be greater when performing sprints on the sand. They also found blood lactate accumulation to be over one and a half times greater during the sand sprints. Of particular significance were the next day performance findings. The researchers found that though the intensities were higher, sprint training on the sand did not lead to a breakdown in next day performance (5).

Sprint training in the sand allowed the athletes to train at higher intensities, allowing for greater gains in aerobic, anaerobic, and lactate threshold capacities. Subsequently the athletes also saw significantly less breakdown in next day performance.

The researchers believed that the lower impact forces associated with the softer sand surface were a factor in the next day performance outcomes. To test this theory, in 2003 a team of researchers out of Japan set out to test the levels of soreness and muscular damage resulting from drop jumping on wood versus sand surfaces. The subjects performed 5 sets of twenty drop jumps, with ten seconds of rest between jumps and two minutes of rest between sets. The researchers then tested Isometric strength and creatine kinase (*a marker of muscle protein breakdown*) 1,24, 36, 48, and 96 hours after the jump session. The researchers found significantly lower markers of muscular damage and lower ratings of muscular soreness in those subjects who performed the drop jumps in the sand (31).

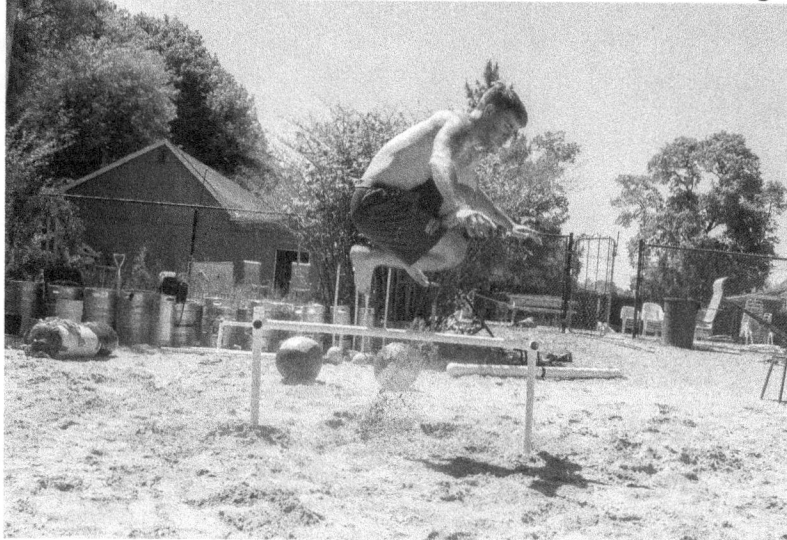

In summary, training in the sand can:

- Dramatically improve balance and agility
- Strengthen stabilizer muscles of ankles, knees, and hips
- Improve core and low back strength
- Correct structural imbalances
- Significantly increase caloric expenditure
- Enhance aerobic, anaerobic, and lactate threshold capacities
- Allow you to train at a higher intensity with less next-day performance breakdown
- Lead to lower levels of muscular damage and soreness

Next let's take a look at sand training methods for enhancing speed, agility, acceleration and jumping ability.

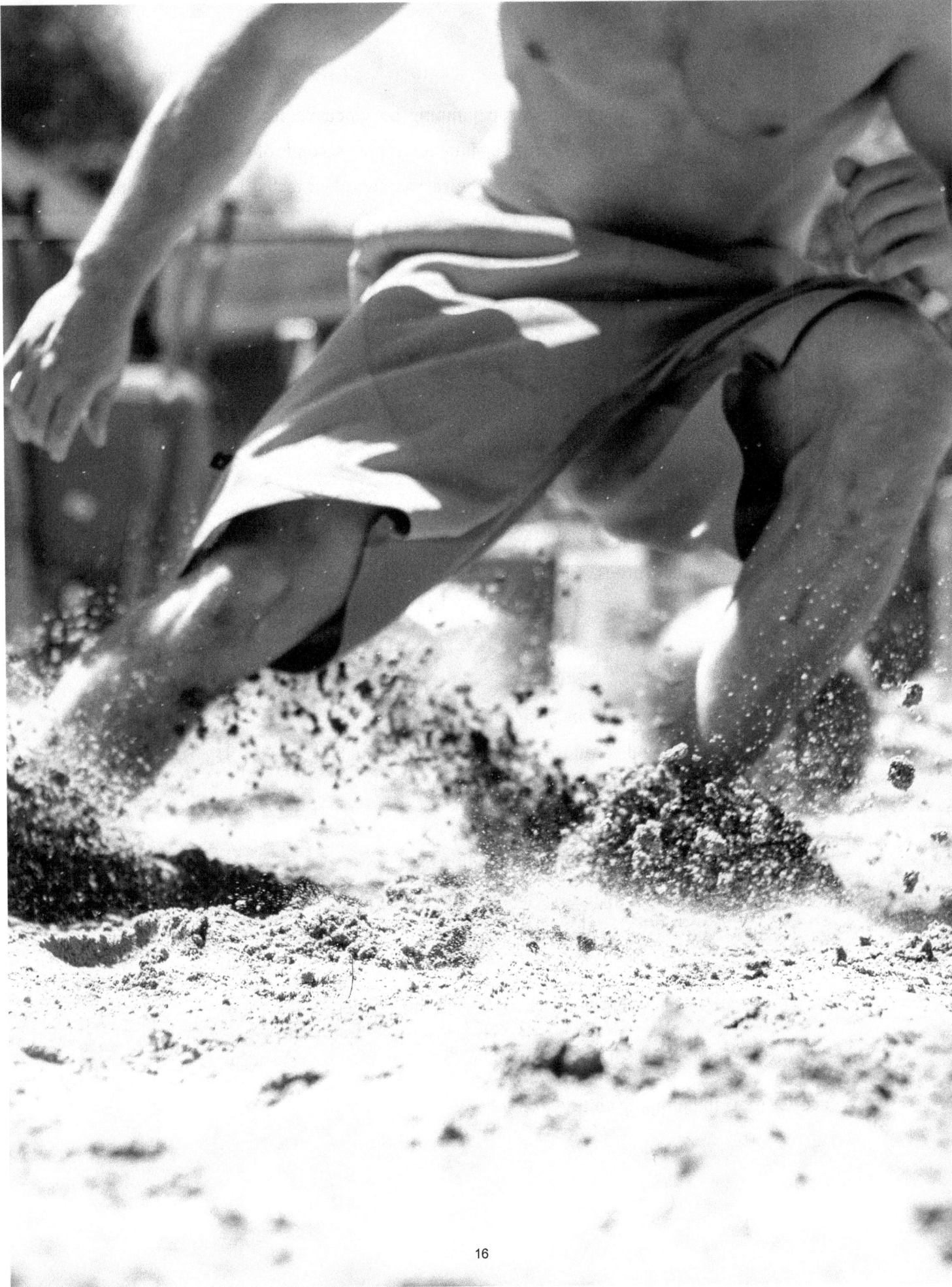

Chapter II

Speed, Agility, and Sand

Speed is the result of several qualities of human performance, including acceleration, strength, elasticity, neuromuscular efficiency, movement quality, flexibility, and more. Great sprinters may not always possess the greatest strength in the weight room. But what they lack in strength, they more than make up for in elasticity, sprint mechanics, movement quality, and range of motion. These athletes look as if they are bouncing of the track with each foot strike. These athletes may take slightly longer to accelerate to full speed, but once there; they may catch and pass the rest of the field.

On the other end of the spectrum are the very strong and very powerful athletes. These athletes including Shot Putters, Olympic Weightlifters, and gymnasts are capable of exploding out of the blocks and accelerating to top speed in a relatively short distance. Often times these athletes will also have impressive vertical or broad jumping ability. In simplest terms, these athletes have tremendous horsepower in their motors. A great example of this strength quality is the Bobsledder. Bobsledders need to push a sled over roughly 50

> **Minimum standards to make Canadian National Bobsled Team (27yrs+):**
> - **Front Squat:** 125kg (F), 200kg (M),
> - **Power Clean:** 100kg (F), 140kg (M)
> - **15m Sprint:** 2.30s (F), 2.15s (M)
> - **30m Sprint:** 4.05s (F), 3.75s (M)
> - **Standing Long Jump:** 2.60m (F), 3.00m (M)
>
> *Keep in mind; these women are roughly 150lbs while men are roughly 200lbs.*
> *From Team Canada Bobsleigh/Skeleton Recruitment Webpage www.bobsleighcanadaskeleton.ca*

meters trying to accelerate it to great enough speeds where it will carry the momentum down through the track.

Then we have the athletes who have a unique combination of both qualities: strength and power to accelerate rapidly or jump through the roof, combined with elasticity, movement quality, and range of motion to achieve higher top speeds. These athletes often perform well in all aspects of speed and acceleration including 5-10-5 pro agility, Illinois Agility Drill, 40-yard dash, and vertical jump.

So where does training in the sand play a role in all of this? Conventional training methods for improving speed that have worked successfully over the years may include weight training, plyometrics, track/field work/practice, hill sprinting, modified strongman training, resisted/assisted sprint training, and soft tissue/flexibility work to name a few. Each of these can be used as tools for improving lagging qualities of speed, agility, acceleration, and jumping ability.

Sand training can be considered a less conventional, yet highly effective method for developing many of these qualities. When performed on the sand, the desired outcomes of many exercises can be magnified due to the greater mechanical and biological demands on the body. According to the research literature, training in the sand can:

- Increase speed through the exaggerated hamstring action during hip extension and the exaggerated gastroc/soleus action during plantar flexion. During acceleration and jumping, as an athlete drives their foot into a hard surface, the surface has no give, creating a reaction force equal to and opposite the ground contact force. When these activities are performed on sand, the surface gives, allowing the foot to drive/slip both downward and backward into the sand, exaggerating the plantar flexion and hip extension movements. This exaggeration of hip extension and plantar flexion leads to a greater training load on the muscles responsible for these movements. Vertical jump can also be increased through this phenomenon.

- Significantly improve total body concentric power as expressed by the squat jump. Sand training has also been shown to improve counter step or elastic jumping ability.

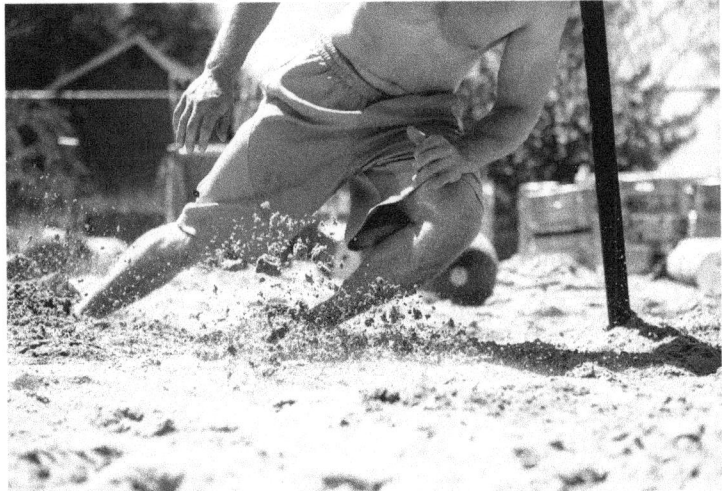

A 2008 study from the *Journal of Sports Medicine* tested the effects of plyometric training 3 times per week for four weeks on either sand or grass. The researchers tested squat and countermovement jumps, 10 and 20m sprints, and level of muscle soreness [24]. The week-to-week breakdown of the workout was as follows:

Exercise	Week 1	Week 2	Week 3	Week 4
Vertical Jumping	15 sets of 10 reps	20 sets of 10 reps	25 sets of 10 reps	25 sets of 10 reps
Bounding	3 sets of 10	4 sets of 10	5 sets of 10	5 sets of 10
Broad Jumping	5 sets of 8	5 sets of 10	7 sets of 10	8 sets of 10
Drop Jump	3 sets of 5	5 sets of 9	6 sets of 15	6 sets of 15

The results of four weeks of either grass or sand training are below:

Test	Grass Group Pre	Grass Group Post	Sand Group Pre	Sand Group Post
Squat Jump	34.0cm	35.8cm	34.3cm	37.8cm
Countermovement Jump	37.8cm	43.3cm	37.2cm	39.6cm

Impellizzeri F, Rampinini E, Castagna C, Martino F, Fiorini S, Wisloff U. **Effect of plyometric training on sand versus grass on muscle soreness and jumping and sprinting ability in soccer players.** *Journal of Sports Medicine.* 42; Pp. 42-46. 2008.

The most significant findings of the study were the comparative gains in squat jump and countermovement jump. The sand training group saw considerably greater gains (3.5cm gain) in the hard surface squat jump test, while the grass training group saw much better gains in the countermovement jump (5.5cm gain), although the sand training group did see a 2.4cm gain in this test. The researchers concluded that the squat jump increases from sand training were due to a combination of greater concentric requirement and less elastic pre-stretch augmentation (24). The greater gains in countermovement jump seen in the grass training group were due to the greater elastic requirements of training on the grass. It is for these reasons that we recommend athletes participate in both hard surface and sand training workouts.

> A 2009 study from the *Journal of Human Sport and Exercise* tested the average squat jump and countermovement vertical jump of 30 elite beach volleyball players (35):
> - **Squat Jump Men:** 44.45cm
> - **Squat Jump Female:** 36.13cm
> - **CMJ Men:** 46.86cm
> - **CMJ Female:** 38.58cm

- Increase speed, acceleration, vertical jump, and agility through the increased demands placed on the stabilizer muscles of the ankles, knees, hips, low back, and core. With greater stability about each joint, movement quality can be improved. When movement quality is improved energy leaks are resolved. This leads to improved efficiency of movement, requiring less energy to perform the same tasks.

- Dramatically improve agility on hard surfaces through improvements in balance, concentric forces, and deceleration efficiency.

- Increase aerobic, anaerobic, and lactate threshold capacity to allow athletes to perform greater number of quality repetitions or sets in a given workout.

The addition of sand training as a training tool in and of itself, can significantly amplify the performance outcomes of various training methodologies. Let's take a brief look at some conventional training methods that have been used successfully for enhancing speed, acceleration, vertical jump, and agility include:

Conventional Strength Training

This is where the horsepower is added to the motor. Along with horsepower, strength training is an effective method for increasing muscular balance, improving movement quality, enhancing body composition and lean muscle tissue, and increasing overall strength. Another significant aspect of strength training is the cascade of positive hormonal events associated with a hard strength training workout.

Conventional strength training exercises include:

Lower Body

Back Squat	Front Squat	Deadlift	Split Squat	Step Fwd. Lunges	Walking Lunges
GHR	Leg Press	Romanian Deadlift	Reverse Hyperextension	Step Up Variations	Hamstring Curl Variations

Torso

Chin Ups	Pull Ups	Row Variations	Pullovers	Lat Pulldowns	Shrugs
Flat Bench Press	Decline Bench Press	Incline Bench Press	Dips	Flyes	Pushups

Arms

Standing Curl Variations	Preacher Curls	Scott Curls	Incline DB Curls	Overhand Curls	Hammer Curls
Dips	French Press	Skull Crushers	Overhead Triceps Extensions	Triceps Pressdowns	Kickbacks

Shoulders, Calves, Abs, Forearms

Standing Overhead Press	Military Press	Upright Rows	Lateral Raises	External Rotator Variations	Trap-3 and Rhomboid Variations
Standing Calf Raise Variations	Seated Calf Raises	Crunch Variations	Leg/Knee Raise Variations	Wrist Curl Variations	Gripping Exercises

Squat Depth

The debate has seemed to rage on for decades. Olympic weightlifters believe in and recommend deep squatting. Powerlifters migrate toward the parallel version. Many doctors and physical therapists are now becoming more aware of the benefits of each. Perhaps squat depth should be an individual preference: what works for you according to what your needs/goals are.

A 2002 study provided valuable insight into squat depth and muscle activation. In this groundbreaking study, the researchers found glute activation during full squat to be greater than twice that of partial squats (35.4% compared to 16.9%), hamstring activation to be similar, while quadriceps activation dominated during the partial squats only (10). Understanding the importance of this can be a critical element in protecting oneself from injury, while achieving desired training outcomes.

Basic biomechanics of the squat consist of hip flexion, knee flexion, dorsiflexion, and spinal pressurization during the eccentric component and hip extension, knee extension, plantar flexion, and spinal pressurization/stability.

A 2012 study from the *Journal of Strength and Conditioning Research* tested the effects deep front squats, deep back squats, and quarter back squats on a Smith Machine had on vertical jump performance. 23 female and 36 male physical education students were broken down into 4 groups and trained for 10 weeks using deep front, deep back, or quarter back squats and the control group. Loading parameters were 8-10 reps for first 4 weeks, 6-8 reps for next 3 weeks, and 2-4 reps for last 3 weeks. The deep front squat saw the biggest gains (over 8% increase) in the countermovement jump and squat jump (over 7%). The deep back squat group had slightly less increases, while the quarter squat group saw minimal gains in both (22).

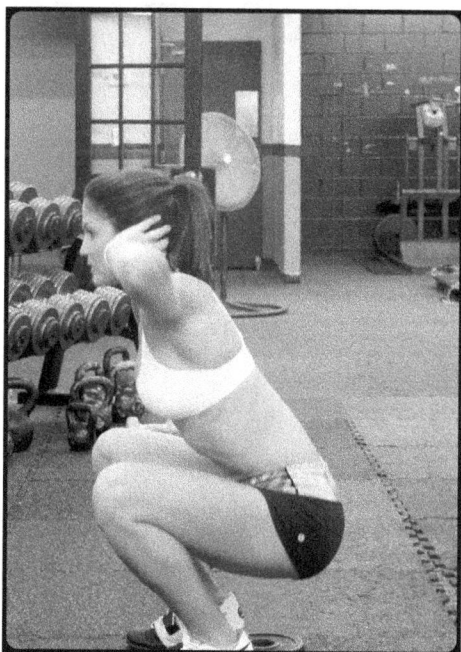

In 2013 a research team out of the Institute of Sports Sciences in Germany and the Australian Institute of Sport thoroughly combed through over 160 scientific research studies or articles relevant to squat technique, depth, and safety (21). After analyzing all of the data they found that:

• "The greatest compressive and retropatellar forces combined with lowest surface contact were found at 90 degrees, while deeper squats were more protective of the knees due to increased surface contact between the quad tendon and intercondylar notch (21).

• Not allowing the knee to travel forward during

the squat can be dangerous as it increases the tensile forces placed on spinal ligaments and shear forces on the intervertebral discs (21).

- Slow tempo during the eccentric phase decreases the shear and compressive forces on the knee joint. 3-4 second eccentric is recommended (21).
- Deep squats do not produce nearly enough shear force on the ACL and PCL to cause any harm. Contrary to popular belief, it was the half squats that were found to produce higher levels of shear force on the ACL (21).

Deep squats have been also been shown in research to increase vertical jump more than half or quarter squats. A 10 week study from 2012 found over an 8% increase in vertical jump after 10 weeks of deep front or back squats. The group that did partial squats saw statistically insignificant gains vertical jump (22).

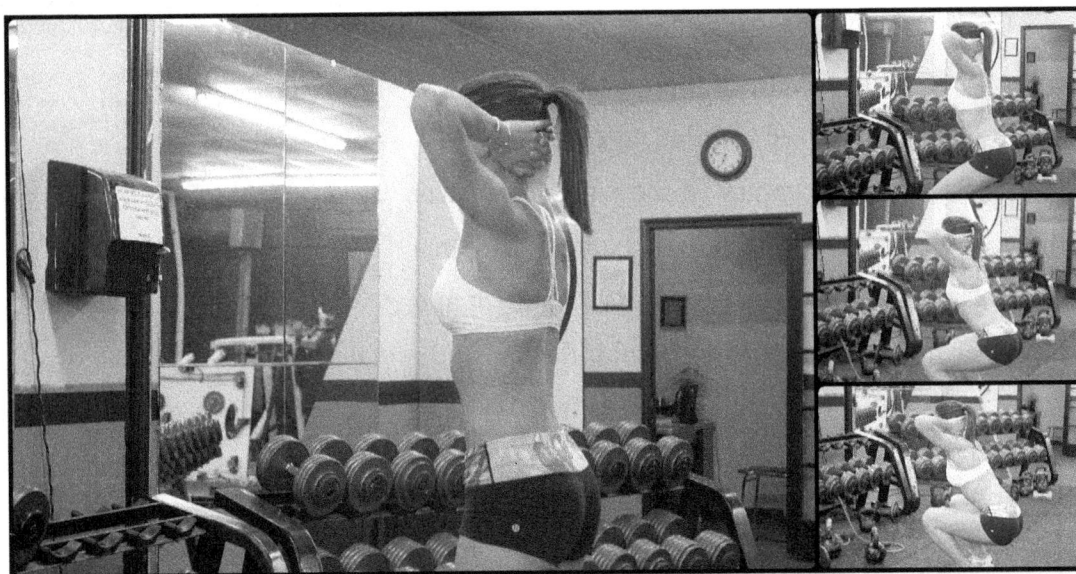

Under the premise that muscles exert their force by pulling on bones we can gain a better understanding of how proper technique deep squatting can actually protective of the knee. "With greater activation/recruitment from a larger number of muscle groups, the knees are better protected during both the eccentric and concentric phases of the motion. For example, in the correct deep squat position (knees pulled out to the sides, slight lean in the torso, lordotic/neutral posture), the adductors on the inside of the thigh and hamstrings on both sides of the knee stabilize the knee to negate the anterior forces of the quadriceps. This combined with greater VMO activation at the bottom 15 degrees of motion and the knee can be kept strong and stable throughout the movement (36)."

The squat to parallel safety dogma appears to draw its roots from a study on knee ligament stability in weightlifters versus non weight lifter. In his study the researcher pre-qualified 128 competitive weightlifters and compared their knee ligament stability to that of 360 non-trained college students (26). Pre-qualifying the subjects may have led to slight research bias, as the ligament stability test was performed with manual force application, rather than a measurable/quantifiable force. The subjects would be pre-qualified (lifter or not) then the testers would determine how much force to apply to their knee structure.

Once the study was made public, and deep squatting was vilified, the news spread like wildfire, and soon deep squats became public enemy number one in the physical therapy and medical communities.

To test the validity of these findings a separate research team reproduced the same study 10 years later. They used the same mediolateral collateral ligament testing instrument to measure ligament stability. Their unbiased findings were quite different. The researchers found no significant differences in collateral ligament instability and knee joint flexibility within any of the squat training groups (30).

"Other studies have had similar findings (11,34). In fact, a study from the *American Journal of Sports Medicine* performed in 1986 compared the knee health of powerlifters to that of college basketball players and 10K recreational runners. The researchers found an increase in posterior/anterior knee laxity in the runner/basketball player group, not the weight training group (39).

Contradictory to popular belief, research has shown that properly executed deep squats (for those with good lower extremity health) do not increase knee laxity/instability, but can actually increase passive tissue health and muscle recruitment, which can lead to increases in performance on the field. So, if deep squats don't cause knee instability than what could some of the possible culprits be? In 1989 a group of researchers tested the knee laxity of 20 recreational long distance runners before and after running. The researchers found an increase in ligamentous laxity post exercise (25)."

Olympic Weightlifting

A staple of many collegiate strength and conditioning programs, Olympic Weightlifting promotes explosive triple extension, similar to biomechanical movement of accelerating and jumping. The Olympic lifts consist of the Snatch and the Clean and Jerk. Modified versions of these exercises are performed from various start or catch positions.

Athletes and strength coaches have used these exercises for decades due to their efficiency, explosive characteristics and ability to develop powerful triple extension. Studies have shown that there is a significant correlation between Olympic Weightlifting performance and 20m-sprint and agility performance [37].

A great quality of Olympic Weightlifting is efficiency. With just one lift, an athlete is able to recruit a high number of muscle fibers. It may be the most compound of compound exercises. The same muscles of the posterior chain used in jumping and sprinted are heavily recruited in the Olympic Lifts. Upon completion of the second pull, the catch involves a deep front or overhead squat (or partial squat in power clean or power snatch), requiring the muscles about the core, back, shoulders, quadriceps, and hips to catch the weight. The athlete is then required to perform a concentric front or overhead squat drive the weight upward.

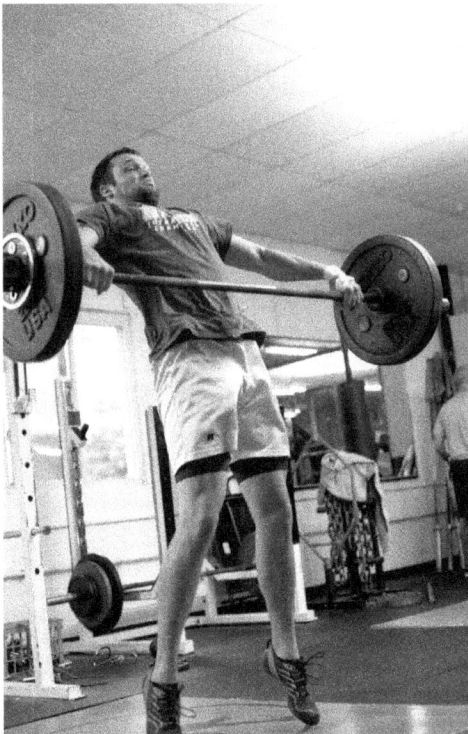

Studies on strength, Olympic Weightlifting performance and their correlation to on field performance have shown that those athletes demonstrating greater abilities in the Olympic lifts and front squat also had more favorable scores in on-field biomarker tests [23,40]. Studies have also shown that the stronger the athlete, the better their performance in the Olympic Lifts [14]."

"In 2008 researchers looked at the short sprint and 5 yard agility performance of Australian Rules football players. The researchers found that those athletes who had better performances in the power clean and front squat also had better scores in the agility and 20m sprints (23). When comparing Olympic Weightlifting to jump training, researchers found that Olympic Weightlifting was the training paradigm that produced a greater transfer for enhancing on field performance markers, in particular increased performance in short burst accelerations (41)."

Not only have Olympic lifts been associated with dramatic increases in strength and power, but their effects on androgenic hormone production are vastly under appreciated. These total body explosive lifts have been shown to have positive effects on androgen hormones and strength gains (14). Olympic lifts are one of the most efficient methods of optimizing ones strength, power and metabolism.

One oft-overlooked element of the Olympic lifts is their ability to create and improve flexibility. From the initial starting position which requires hamstring flexibility and low back mobility, to the catch which requires flexibility about the hips, shoulders, and back, these lifts are an excellent method of actively training flexibility (37)."

Plyometrics

During the days of Eastern Bloc Olympic dominance, the Soviet teams were supposedly using top secret training methods to create world and Olympic champions. Some U.S. coaches were invited to the Soviet Union to observe these secret training methods.

What they saw were athletes jumping onto and off of platforms, pushing against walls on swing like devices, throwing weights into the air from many different positions, jumping up and grabbing targets suspended from the ceiling, and many other secret training methods. Many of these movements had one thing in common: explosive movement.

Yuri Verkoshansky termed what these coaches were witnessing "shock training". Excited, these coaches went back to the U.S. and began incorporating these methods, many of which became known as "Plyometrics".

Plyometrics in the U.S. seemed to evolve from the original "shock training" to any type of jump training. Eventually anything involved with jumping seemed to fall under the plyometric umbrella. Then, the "more is better" mentality began to slowly creep in, and sub maximal Plyometrics were born. According to the late Mel Siff, for an exercise to be a true (maximal) plyometric exercise it must meet the following 5 criteria [38]:

1. "**Initial Momentum Phase:** This is the initial movement of the body or body parts.

2. **Electromechanical Delay Phase:** (Eccentric Contraction) This is the time delay between motor nerve excitation and actual muscle contraction when contact is made against an immovable surface.

3. **Amortization Phase:** (Isometric Contraction) The phase in which the movement rapidly switches from eccentric to concentric muscle contraction. There is a stretch reflex that occurs in the musculotendinous unit similar to the stretching or mechanical deformation of a trampoline as you land on the surface.

4. **Rebound Phase:** (Concentric Contraction) This is the release of the energy, or the rebound force generated from the stretch reflex. As in the trampoline example, once full stretch has been reached, the elastic energy then accelerates upward in the opposite direction (release of kinetic energy).

5. **Final Momentum Phase:** (Excluding Depth Drops) Once the concentric contraction is complete the body will continue to move because of the release of the elastic energy and force generated from the concentric contraction [38]".

Jump training in the sand cannot be qualified as truly plyometric in nature as it does not meet the above criteria. The amortization phase is too long. The forgivingness of the sand surface allows for the ground contact forces to be dispersed into the ground. The energy is released into the ground rather than used to create an equal and opposite rebound effect. This increases ground contact time, decreases elastic stretch reflex, and increases concentric muscle action demands.

From the criteria provided by Siff, the terms maximal and sub maximal can be used to distinguish between different types of plyometric activity. Maximal

Plyometrics include depth drops and depth jumps. Sub maximal Plyometrics include low cone jumps, low box jumping, low squat jumps, ankle hops, skater hops, etc.

Complex Training

Complex training involves a phenomenon known as post activation potentiation (PAP). "Post activation potentiation is a training phenomenon in which a trainee is capable of potentiating their nervous system to achieve a higher level of activation. In theory this leads to an enhanced motor unit and muscle fiber recruitment during the ensuing event.

The basic theory is to acutely enhance nervous system and muscular force output. This is done by performing a heavy, high threshold muscle fiber recruitment exercise, and follow it with an explosive movement that requires similar musculature.

A 2010 study out of the *Journal of Strength and Conditioning Research* studied the effects three different conditioning stimuli (3 rep max half squat, plyo, and inactivity) had on jumping ability. What they found was that after a five minute rest period, the subjects whom performed the 3 rep max half squats saw more favorable results in the countermovement jump height than plyometric exercises or rest [13].

In a separate study out of the Neuromuscular Laboratory at Appalachian State University, researchers compared the effects stimulatory effects heavy squats, loaded countermovement jumps, or rest had on 10, 30, and 40m sprint performance in college football players. After performing the stimulatory exercise followed by four minutes of rest, the subjects who performed the heavy squats first realized the best performances in the 10, 30, and 40m sprints, especially in those subjects whom were characterized as weaker per pound of body weight [28].

Examples of Post Activation Training utilizing a combination of conventional and sand training methods include:

Example 1

Exercise	Reps	Sets	Tempo	Rest Interval
A1: Barbell Back Squat With Chains	3	6	30X1	30s
A2: 2 Legged Broad Jump in the sand	1	6	NA	120s

Example 2

Exercise	Reps	Sets	Tempo	Rest Interval
A1: Front Squat	2-3	5	32X1	30s
A2: 10m Sand Sprint from 40 start position	1	5	NA	120s

Example 3

Exercise	Reps	Sets	Tempo	Rest Interval
A1: Rack Pull	3	6	21X1	30s
A2: Overhead Goal Vertical Jump on sand	1	6	NA	120s

Example 4

Exercise	Reps	Sets	Tempo	Rest Interval
A1: Clean High Pull	3	6	X0X0	30s
A2: Standing Triple Jump in the sand	1	6	NA	120s

Example 5

Exercise	Reps	Sets	Tempo	Rest Interval
A1: Fat Grip Barbell Bench Press with chains	3	6	30X0	30s
A2: Hand Over Hand Atlas Stone Push	10 Yards	6	NA	120s

Example 6

Exercise	Reps	Sets	Tempo	Rest Interval
A1: 10 Yard Super Yoke	1	8	NA	30s
A2: 15 Yard Bounding in the sand	15yds	8	NA	120s

Functional Strength Training

Strongman training can be a great method for improving functional strength and hypertrophy. It is a very effective training method for bridging the gap between weight room and on-field importance. When performed properly, strongman training can:

- Increase lower back and posterior chain strength
- Increase core strength in an upright position

- Strengthen the VMO musculature during the eccentric loading element of walking exercises
- Increase ankle stability
- Increase grip strength
- Strengthen connective tissue
- Have positive effects on bone density
- Increase neuromuscular efficiency of synergistic muscles involved in upright stability
- Increase functional strength of the hip flexors and extensors
- Increase musculotendinous strength of the elbow flexors
- Increase lactic and alactic capacity
- Build mental toughness....

No longer a training method reserved for 300+ pound strongmen, modified versions of this training modality have firmly implanted their roots into mainstream training methodology. Large commercial health clubs have added variations of strongman training including sandbag carrying, farmer carries, sled drags, hand over hand rope pulls, and tire flipping. Elite performance training centers geared toward the highest level of athletics utilize many of the above in conjunction with proper programming to create a foundation for optimal athletic performance.

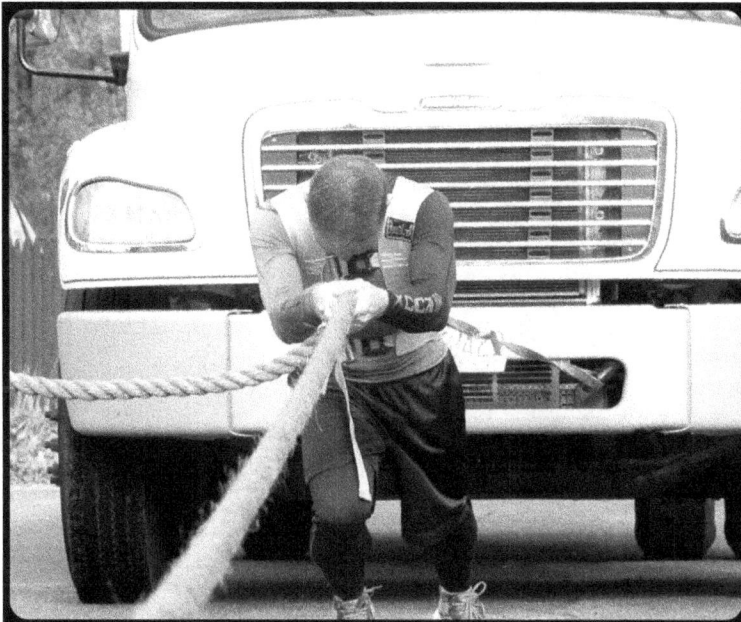

Strongman training is functional training in its purest form. By focusing on non-isolated, multi-segmental movements, the transfer effect to the field can be very high.

The activity of core musculature is greater in strongman exercises than most core specific exercises. While the abdominals do play a role in upright stabilization, it is the co-activation of the abdominal, oblique and erector spinae musculature that creates the intra-abdominal pressurization that leads to enhanced spinal stability [29]. Lifts such as squats and deadlifts have also been shown to have significantly greater core activation than the popular isometric plank hold [20].

Without abdominal/oblique, hip, and spinal erector co-activation, upright stability may be compromised. By focusing their efforts on standing, load bearing, and preferably dynamic movements, athletes can achieve highly transferable results from their hard training.

A 2009 study set out to establish the trunk musculature activation of Strongman training modalities. The researchers found tremendous supporting evidence toward the usage of upright loaded strongman exercises and transferable activation of the "core" musculature [29].

In this study, peak muscle activation of the rectus abdominis, internal and external obliques was found in all of the events, but was found to be **highest in the walking phase of the Farmer Walk, Super Yoke Walk, and the Suitcase Carry** [4]. A separate study from 2007 had similar findings with regards to trunk activation and object holding/carrying. 11 male subjects had to walk between 1.9 and 3.3 mph while carrying a barbell at 3 different heights and then a bucket of potatoes at 3 different heights. The researchers found 33%, 49%, and 47% increase in erector spinae musculature in the walking barbell group versus the standing barbell group. **The walking group also had a 51% and 65% greater activation in the rectus abdominis and external oblique when compared to standing Group** [1]. Of even greater significance was the abdominal

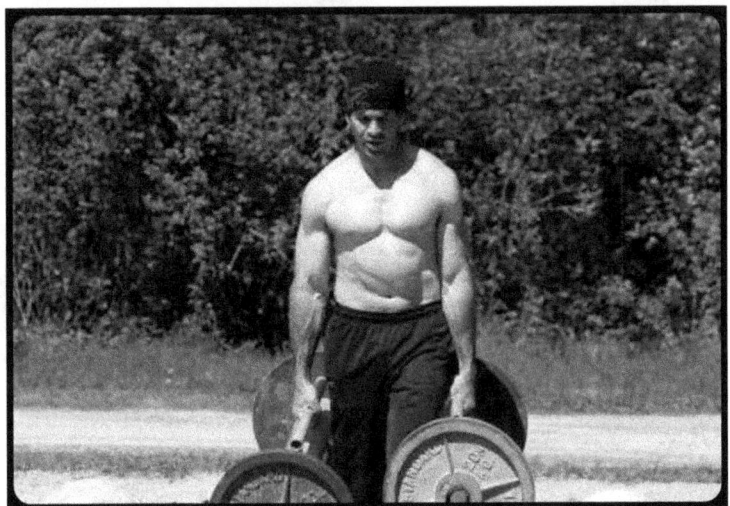

activity of the group walking with the bucket of potatoes. The researchers found a ***132% increase in rectus abdominis activity in the walking group compared with the standing group*** (1). When walking with the bucket at knuckle or elbow height there was a two fold increase in rectus abdominis activity (1).

While Strongman training is a great tool for enhancing on field physicality, some elements may not be appropriate on soft sand surfaces, while others may me just downright sadistic. For example, tire flipping, Super Yoke, and Atlas stone loading may be safer and better suited for solid surfaces.

On the other hand, farmer carries, keg carries, keg throws, kettlebell throws, sled drags, hand over hand rope pulls, and throwing events are made considerably more difficult with the instability of the sand surface.

For example the farmer carry on a solid surface is a great exercise for strengthening the muscles about the ankles, knees, hips, low back and muscles about the shoulder girdle. It also strengthens knee stability through the eccentric load it places on the VMO muscle with each foot strike.

Taking this exercise into the sand can dramatically amplify the stability requirements of the entire kinetic chain from ankles to shoulders. Adding slalom style directional changes can increase these demands to an even greater extent.

Sprint Training Variations

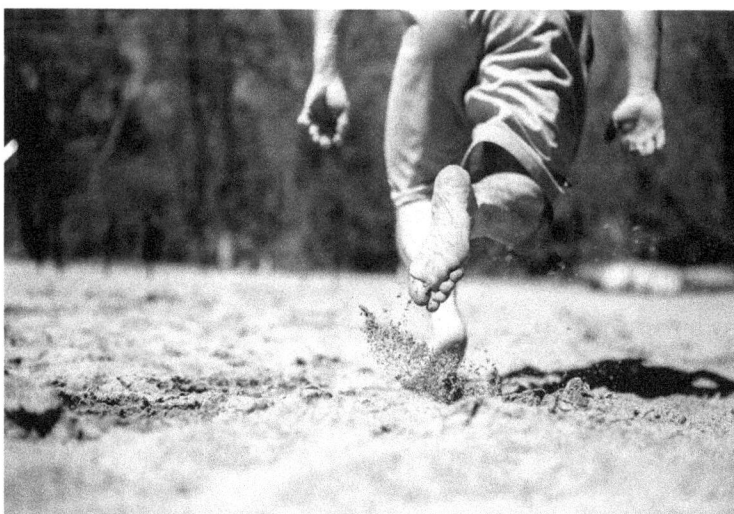

Sprint training can be an effective method of building top speed, acceleration, leg strength, elastic elements of the lower extremities, lower body hypertrophy, lactate and alactic capacity, and general conditioning. Different sprint modalities include:

- **Short sprints** to improve acceleration. 5, 10, 15, 20 yard sprints from a variety of different start positions are examples.
- **5-10-5 pro agility** and **Illinois drill** for acceleration, deceleration, and change of direction.
- **Moderate distance sprints** of 30-60 yards to improve alactic capacity and the ability to accelerate to top speed.
- **Resisted sprint training** in the form of light sleds, parachutes, and other devices are used to improve acceleration and condition. These devices can also be used as conditioning tools. Autoregulatory 15m resisted sprints can be an effective training tool for enhancing acceleration.

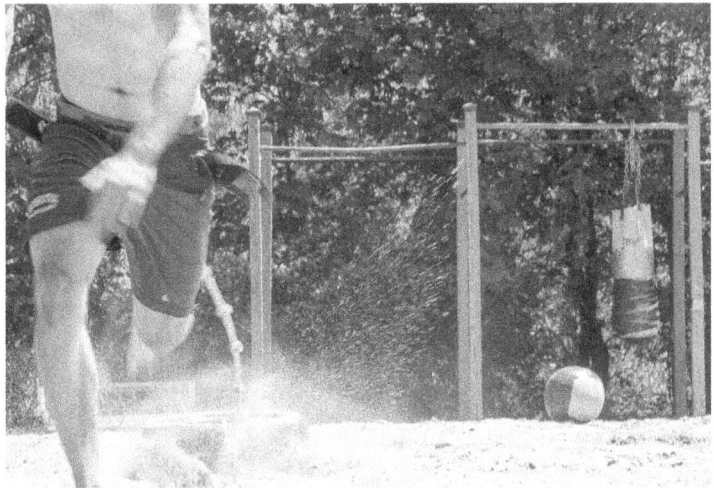

- **80's:** One of our favorites. This is the modified version of the concepts learned from the Boston College football strength coach when BC was recognized as one of the fittest teams in college football. Depending on the age and position, athletes have somewhere between 8 and 11 seconds to sprint 80 yards. During the first week they are running 3-4 of these and have 45 seconds to get back to start. By the end of the summer, the athletes are running between 20-32 (broken into blocks of 5 or 8 then 120s rest) of these sprints, with 30-35s of recovery between sprints.
- **Autoregulatory Sprints**: Quality training over quantity training. Athlete will run their best timed sprint. For example the athlete runs a 4.7 40 yard dash. The athlete is then allowed a 3-5% drop off in performance in the ensuing sprints. In this case once the athlete cannot run consecutive 40's in less than 4.935s (5% drop off of 4.7) they are done due to a decrease in the quality of work.
- **Long sprints** to build lactate capacity and general conditioning. Anything over 80 yards up to 400m.

- **Hill sprints** are a great way to develop the hip extensor musculature while minimizing impact forces. Caution should be taken to avoid Achilles tendon issues during hill sprint protocols.
- **Sand to hard surface sprints:** Start 5-10 yards in the sand then sprint out of the sand and continue sprint for pre-determined distance on hard surface.
- **Fartlek Training** for improved conditioning. Sprint for a pre-determined time or distance, then active recovery for pre-determined time or distance.

As we saw earlier performing many of these on the sand can increase the mechanical workload, decrease the risk of injury, and improve sprint performance. A training programme consisting of both sand and field/track sprint protocols is recommended. The harder surface allows for greater gains in the elastic elements associated with sprinting, while the sand requires greater concentric action, energy expenditure, and mechanical work.

A 2013 study from the *Journal of Science and Sports Medicine* may have summed up best the increased energy demand of sand sprinting when they concluded *"These results show that on sand it is possible to perform maximal intensity sprints with higher energy expenditure and metabolic power values, without reaching maximum speed and with smaller impact shocks. Furthermore, exercises with change of direction carried out on this surface allow participants to reach higher deceleration values (15)."*

Cone and Agility Ladder Drills

These drills are by coaches and athletes to potentially improve agility and quickness.

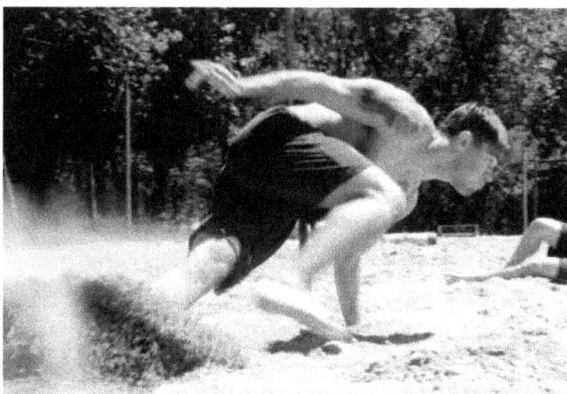

As many of these drills are learnable patterns, the transfer to on field performance may not be as high some of the aforementioned training methods. When performed on sand, though, the unstable surface will amplify the mechanical work, stabilizer activity, and caloric expenditure. Drills include:

- **Zig zag** and **slalom cone drills**: When performed in the sand, the increased neuromuscular demands can enhance balance, lower extremity strength, and upright stability.
- **5-10-5** and **Illinois Drill** on the sand. Increased eccentric and concentric demands during the acceleration and deceleration components.
- **Agility Ladder Drills**: the sand adds to the mechanical demands and can dramatically increase the difficulty of these patterns.

As can be seen, there are many methods for enhancing athletic performance. By focusing on a foundation of strength, movement quality, and structural balance, athletes create a stable platform upon which gains in speed, power, agility, body composition, and injury management are built. When many of these methods are combined with the instability provided by a soft sand surface, the positive results can be further magnified.

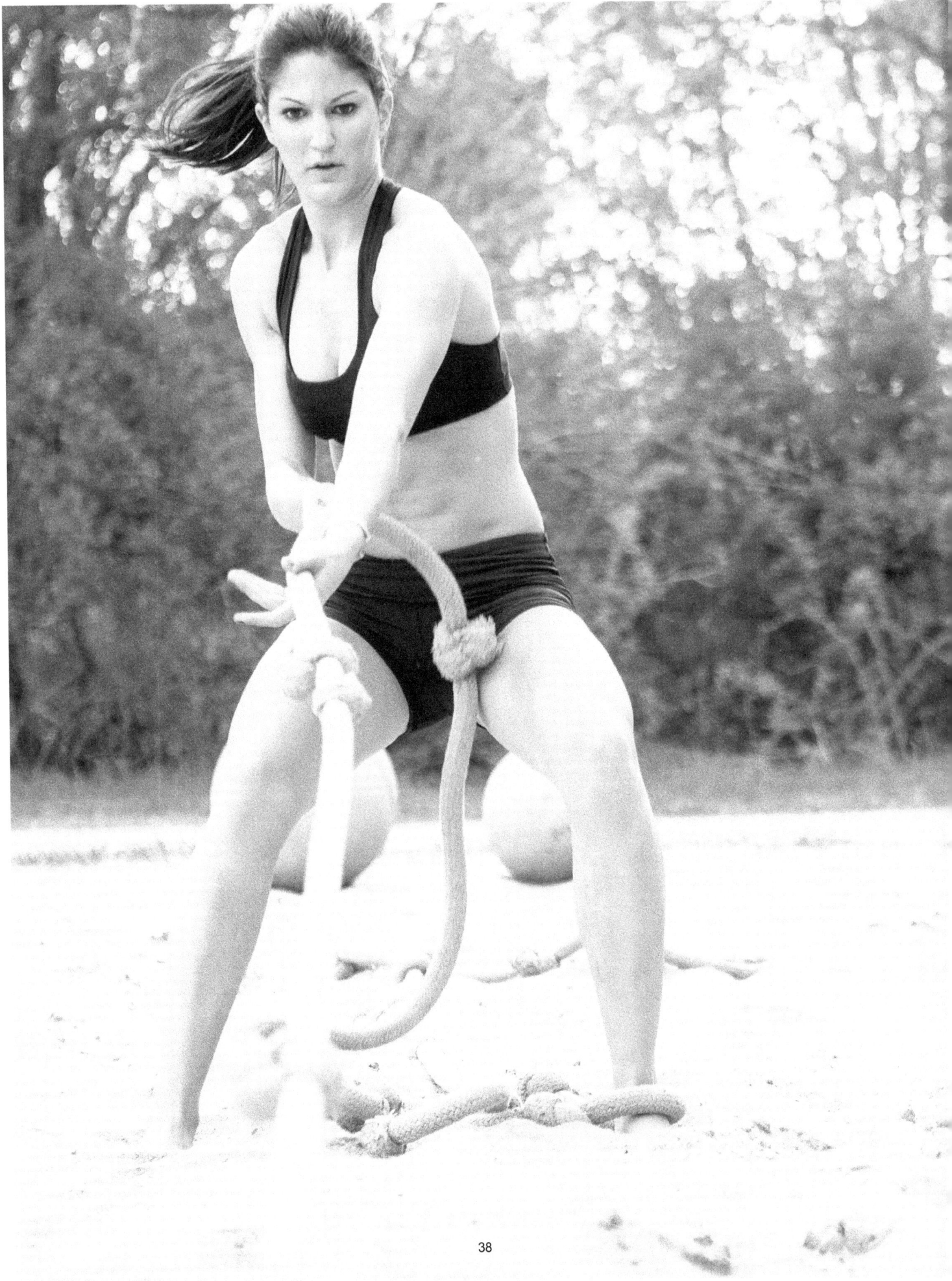

Chapter III
Programming and Sand Workouts

Similar to the squat depth debate, programming and periodization that works well for one individual may not work as well for another. Let's briefly discuss a few periodization paradigms and then delve into programming concepts.

Common periodization models include:

- **Linear Periodization:** Progressive form of periodization in which progression occurs in a linear fashion in which each phase emphasizes a specific training quality, eventually building up to physical peak. Example of 16 week linear periodization:

Week	Weeks 1-4	Weeks 5-8	Weeks 9-12	Weeks 13-16
Phase	Structural Balance	Hypertrophy	Strength	Power
Rep Ranges:	10-12, 12-15	6-8, 7-9, 8-10, 10-12	1-5	1-5
Sets:	3-5/exercise, 20-26 total sets	3-10/exercise, 20-26 total sets	5-10/exercise. 20-32 total sets	5-10/exercise, 20-32 total sets
Tempo:	5010, 4020, 3030, 3010, etc.	4121, 3211, 5050, 3132	31X1, 3011, 2010, 24X1	XOXO
Rest Interval:	45-60s	45-90s	90-180s	90-240s

Linear periodization structural balance phase weekly schedule with sand training:

Monday	Tuesday	Wednesday	Thursday	Friday	Sat	Sun
A1: FFE DB Split Squats X 10-12 @ 4120 X 4sets	Sand Workout Dynamic Warm Up in **Sand**	**A1:** DB Squats X 10-12 @ 4120 X 4sets	Sand Workout Dynamic Warm Up in **Sand**	**Wednesday** **A1:** Walking Lunges X 10-12 @ 4120 X 4sets	Rest or Yoga	Rest or Yoga
A2: Standing DB Overhead press X 10-12@ 3010 X 4 sets	**A:** Low Hurdle Hops in **sand** X 5 reps 60-90s rest X 5 sets	**A2:** Incline DB Bench Press X 10-12@ 3010 X 4 sets	**A:** Lateral Hurdle Hops in **sand** X 6 reps 60-90s rest X 5 sets	**A2:** Dips X 10-12@ 3010 X 4 sets		
B1: Box Step Ups X 10-12@ 1010 X 4 sets **B2:** Chin Ups X 10-12 @ 3210 X 4 sets	**B:** Depth Drops in **sand** X 10 total reps 30-90s rest between reps	**B1:** Kneeling Hamstring Curls X 6-8 @ 4022 X 4 sets **B2:** Seated Cable Rows X 10-12 @ 3012 X 4 sets	**B:** Overhead Goal Counter Step Jumps in **sand** 2reps X 6 sets 30-90s rest between sets	**B1:** Swiss Ball Hamstring Curls X 6-8 @ 4022 X 4 sets **B2:** Ring Inverted Rows X 10-12 @ 3012 X 4 sets		
C1: Low Back Extensions X 10-12 @ 3011 X 4 sets	**C:** T Test in the **sand** X 6 sets 60-120s rest between sets	**C1:** Reverse Hyperextensions X 10-12 @ 3011 X 4 sets	**C:** Illinois Drill in the **sand** X 6 sets 60-120s rest between sets	**C1:** Landmine X 10-12 @ 3011 X 4 sets		
C2: Overhead Cable Triceps Extensions X 10-12 @ 3010 X 4 sets **C3:** Seated DB Curls X 10-12 @ 3010 X 4 sets	**D:** 5-10-20 yd shuttle sprint in the **sand** X 6 sets 60-120s rest between sets	**C2:** Triceps Pressdowns X 10-12 @ 3010 X 4 sets **C3:** Preacher Curls X 10-12 @ 3010 X 4 sets	**D:** Sand to hard surface sprint X 30 yds. (10yds sand/20yds hard surface) X 6 sets 60-120s rest	**C2:** Close Grip Pushups X 10-12 @ 3010 X 4 sets **C3:** Fat Grip Barbell Curls X 10-12 @ 3010 X 4 sets		
D1: Seated Cable External Rotator X 10-12 @ 3011 X 2 sets **D2:** Face Pulls X 10-12 @ 3011 X 2 Sets	**E1:** Hand Over Hand Atlas Stone Push Slalom X 20 yds. X 6 sets 15s rest **E2:** Farmer Carry Slalom in **sand** X 20 Yards X 6 sets 120-180s rest	**D1:** Standing Cable External Rotator X 10-12 @ 3011 X 2 sets **D2:** 2 Arm Trap-3 Lift X 10-12 @ 3011 X 2 Sets	**E1:** Hand Over Hand Atlas Stone Pull X 20 yds. X 6 sets 15s rest **E2:** Overhead Slosh Stick Carry in **sand** X 20 yds. X 6 sets 120-180s rest	**D:** Cuban Press X 10-12 @ 3011 X 2 sets		

- **Undulating Periodization:** Periodization method that involves training variation throughout the week. Specific training qualities are emphasized on separate workouts days (daily undulating) or weeks (weekly undulating). An example of a daily undulating periodization model may look like this:

Weeks 1-4	Day 1	Day 2	Day 3
Emphasis	Strength	Structural Balance	Hypertrophy
Rep Ranges:	1-5	10-12, 12-15	6-8, 7-9, 8-10, 10-12
Sets:	5-10/exercise. 20-32 total sets	3-5/exercise, 20-26 total sets	3-10/exercise, 20-26 total sets
Tempo:	31X1, 3011, 2010, 24X1	5010, 4020, 3030, 3010, etc.	4121, 3211, 5050, 3132
Rest Interval:	90-180s	45-60s	45-90s

Undulating periodization structural balance phase weekly schedule with sand training:

Monday	Tuesday	Wednesday	Thursday	Friday	Sat	Sun
A1: Front Squat X 3-5 @ 3210 X 6sets **A2:** Prone Hamstring Curls X 3-5 @ 3010 X 6 sets **B1:** Fat Grip Barbell Bench Press X 3-5 @ 3010 X 6 sets **B2:** Chin Ups X 3-5 @ 3210 X 6 sets **C1:** Standing Overhead Log Press X 3-5 @ 1012 X 4 sets **C2:** Overhead Cable Triceps Extensions X 3-5 @ 2011 X 4 sets **C3:** Standing Fat Grip Barbell Curls X 3-5 @ 3010 X 4 sets **D1:** Seated Cable External Rotator X 6-8 @ 3011 X 2 sets **D2:** Face Pulls X 6-8 @ 3011 X 2 Sets	**Sand Workout** Dynamic Warm Up in **Sand** **A:** 2-Legged Bounding in **sand** X 20 yds. 60-90s rest X 5 sets **B:** Overhead Goal CMJ in the **sand** X 2 reps 60-90s rest X 5 sets **C:** 5-10-5 Pro Agility in the **sand** X 6 sets 60-120s rest **D1:** Overhead Kettlebell Throws in the sand X 5 reps 20s rest X 5 sets **D2:** 2 Hand Atlas Stone Push X 10 reps 90-120s rest X 5 sets **E1:** Low Crawl in the **sand** X 25 yds. 0-10s rest X 5 sets **E2:** Heavy Bag Carry in the **sand** X 30 Yards X 5 sets 120-180s rest	**A1:** FFE DB Split Squats X 10-12 @ 4020 X 4sets **A2:** Seated DB Overhead press X 10-12@ 3010 X 4 sets **B1:** Single Leg Swiss Ball Hamstring Curls X 6-8 @ 4021 X 4 sets **B2:** Pull-ups X 4-6 @ 3521 X 4 sets **C1:** Kneeling Landmine X 10-12 @ 3011 X 4 sets **C2:** Triceps Pressdowns X 10-12 @ 3010 X 4 sets **C3:** Seated DB Curls X 10-12 @ 3010 X 4 sets **D1:** Standing Cable External Rotator X 10-12 @ 3011 X 2 sets **D2:** Standing Cable Scap Retraction X 5-6 @ 2012 X 2 Sets	**Sand Workout** Dynamic Warm Up in **Sand** **A:** Bounding in **sand** X 20 yds. 60-90s rest X 5 sets **B1:** Forward Underhand Kettlebell Throws in the **sand** X 3-5 with 30s of rest X 6 sets **B2:** Broad Jump in the **sand** X2 with 60-120s rest X 6 sets **C:** Illinois Drill in the **sand** X 6 sets 60-120s rest between sets **D: Sand** to hard surface sprint X 30 yds. (10yds **sand**/20yds hard surface) X 6 sets 60-120s rest **E1:** Hand Over Hand Atlas Stone Pull X 20 yds. X 6 sets 15s rest **E2:** Overhead Slosh Stick Carry in sand X 20 yds. X 6 sets 120-180s rest	**Wednesday** **A:** Deadlift X 6-8 @ 3031 X 5sets **B1:** Step Forward Lunges X 8-10 @ 3010 X 4 sets **B2:** Incline DB Bench Press X 8-10 @ 3111 X 4 sets **C1:** Leg Press X 20-25 @ 2010 X 4 sets **C2:** Seated Cable Rows X 8-10 @ 3010 X 4 sets **D1:** Fat Grip Incline DB Curls X 8-10 @ 3010 X 4 sets **D2:** Cable French Press X 8-10 @ 3011 X 4 sets	Rest or Yoga	Rest or Yoga

- **Alternating Phases of Accumulation and Intensification:** A model proposed and implemented with great success by coaches around the globe, including world renowned strength guru, Coach Charles Poliquin. This model of periodization involves alternating between phases of Hypertrophy/Functional Hypertrophy/Structural Balance and Relative Strength training. The concept is that in order to make gains in strength and hypertrophy an athlete needs to alternate between methods that induce sarcoplasmic and myofibrillar hypertrophy.

Sample week including sand training workouts

Monday	Tuesday	Wednesday	Thursday	Fri	Saturday	Sun
A1: Front Squat X 4-6 @ 3210 X 6sets **A2:** Prone Hamstring Curls X 6-8 @ 3012 X 6 sets **B1:** Step Forward Lunges X 8-10 @ 4020 X 5 sets **B2:** Box Step Ups X 8-10 @ 1010 X 5 sets **C1:** Prowler Push X 30yds X 4 sets rest 10s **C2:** Backward Sled Drag X 30 yds. X 4 sets rest 60-90s	**A1:** Neutral Grip Chin Ups X 6-8 @ 3210 X 6sets **A2:** Fat Grip Incline Barbell Bench Press X 6-8 @ 3011 X 6 sets **B1:** Bent Over Barbell Rows X 6-8 @ 3021 X 5 sets **B2:** Ring Dips X 6-8 @ 3011 X 5 sets **C1:** 30 Degree Incline DB Flyes X 10-12 @ 3010 X 4 Sets **C2:** Face Pulls X 10-12 @ 3010 X 4 Sets	**Sand Workout** Dynamic Warm Up in **Sand** **A:** 2-Legged Bounding in **sand** X 20 yds. 60-90s rest X 5 sets **B:** Overhead Goal CMJ in the **sand** X 2 reps 60-90s rest X 5 sets **C:** 6 cone 5yds apart agility slalom in **sand** X 1 60-90s rest X 8 sets **D1:** Hand Over Hand Rope Pull in **sand** X 20 yds. rest 10s X 5 sets **D2:** 2 Hand Atlas Stone Push X 20 yds. 90-120s rest X 5 sets	**A1:** V-Bar Dips X 6-8 @ 3112 X 5sets **A2:** Preacher Curls X 6-8 @ 3030 X 4 sets **B1:** French Press X 6-8 @ 3121 X 5 sets **B2:** Incline DB Curls X 6-8 @ 3121 X 5 sets **D1:** Standing Cable External Rotator X 10-12 @ 3011 X 2 sets **D2:** Single Arm DB Trap-3 lift X 10-12 @ 3021 X 2 Sets	Off or Yoga	**Sand Workout** Dynamic Warm Up in **Sand** **A1:** Tire Flips on Hard Surface X 2-4 rest 30s 6 sets **A2:** Broad Jump in the sand X 2 at 90-120s rest X 6 sets **B1:** Super Yoke on hard surface X 20 yds. rest 30s X 6 sets **B2:** Bounding in sand X 15 yds. with 90-120s rest X 6 sets **C:** T Drill in the sand X 6 sets 60-120s rest between sets **D1:** Keg Carry Slalom X 30 yds. rest 10s X 5 sets **D2:** Hand Over Hand Atlas Stone Push Slalom X 30yds rest 90-120s X 5 sets **E1:** Hand Over Hand Atlas Stone Pull X 20 yds. X 6 sets 15s rest **E2:** Overhead Slosh Stick Carry X 20 yds. X 6 sets 120-180s rest	

- **Conjugate Method:** Based on the Russian Conjugate method and the programming genius of Louie Simmons, variations of this periodization model have been used with tremendous success to build some of the strongest athletes in the world. An example of a one week Conjugate method of periodization may look like this:

Weeks 1-4	Day 1	Day 2	Day 3	Day 4
Emphasis	Max Effort Lower Body	Max Effort Upper Body	Dynamic Effort Lower Body	Dynamic Effort Upper Body
Rep Ranges:	1-3	1-3	1-3	1-3
Sets:	N for max effort lift, 3-5/exercise for auxiliary work. 20-32 total sets	N for max effort lift, 3-5/exercise for auxiliary work. 20-32 total sets	10 for main lift, 3-5 for auxiliary work, 20-32 total sets	10 for main lift, 3-5 for auxiliary work, 20-32 total sets
Tempo:	Controlled tempo	Controlled tempo	Explosive	Explosive
Rest Interval:	120-300s	120-300s	45-75s	N or 45-60s

Sample Conjugate Training Week including sand training

Monday	Tuesday	Wednesday	Thursday	Friday	Saturday	Sun
A: Max Effort Back Squat X 1-3 @ 3010 rest 120-300s X N sets **B:** Romanian Deadlift X 3-5 @ 2010 rest 60s X 5 sets **C1:** GHR X 4-6 @3010 rest 45s X 5 sets **C2:** Reverse Hyperextensions X 4-6 @ 3010 rest 90s X 5 sets **C1:** Prowler Push X 30yds X 4 sets rest 10s **C2:** Backward Sled Drag X 30 yds. X 4 sets rest 60-90s	**A:** Max Effort Barbell Bench Press X 1-3 @ 3010 rest 120-300s X N sets **B1:** Chin Ups X 3-5 @ 2010 rest 60s X 5 sets **B2:** Parallel Bar Dips X 3-5 @ 2010 rest 90s X 5 sets **C1:** Standing Overhead Log Press X 3-5 @ 2010 rest 60s X 4 Sets **C2:** Fat Grip Triceps Pressdowns X 4-6 @ 2010 rest 90s X 4 Sets **D1:** Seated DB External Rotator X 8-10 @ 3010 rest 30s X 3 sets **D2:** Face Pulls X 8-10 @ 2011 rest 30s X 3 sets	**Sand Workout** Dynamic Warm Up in **Sand** **A:** Overhead Kettlebell Throws in **sand** X 5 rest 60-90s X 5 sets **B:** Chest Pass Med Ball Throws X 5 reps rest 60-90s X 5 sets **C1:** Farmer Carry in **sand** X 20 yds. rest 30s X 5 sets **C2:** Box Squat to broad jump in **sand** X 2 rest 60-90s X 5 sets **D:** Illinois Drill in the **sand** X 1 rest 60s X 6 sets **E:** 30 yd **sand** to hard surface sprint (start 10 yards sand then 20 yards hard surface) X 1 rest 60s X 6 sets	**A1:** Power Clean X 2-4 @ X0X0 rest 120-240s X 6 sets **B1:** Dynamic Squat with Chains X 3 @ 10X0 rest 30s X 5 sets **B2:** Kneeling Hamstring Curl X 3-5 @ 20X0 rest 90s X 5 sets **D1:** Tire Flips X 2 rest 0s X 5 sets **D2:** Backward Sled Drag 20yds rest 0s X 5 Sets **D3:** Tire Flips X 2 rest 0s X 5 sets **D4:** Backward Sled Drag 20yds rest 120-240s X 5 sets	**A1:** Dynamic Fat Grip Bench Press with Chains X 3 @ 10X0 rest 60s X 10 sets **A2:** Bent Over Barbell Rows X 3 @ 2010 rest 60s X 10 sets **B1:** Flat DB Bench Press X 6-8 @ 2010 rest 45s X 3 sets **B2:** Neutral Grip Chin Ups X 6-8 @ 2010 rest 90s X 3 sets **C1:** Seated DB Overhead Press X 6-8 @ 2010 rest 45s X 3 sets **C2:** Standing Cable External Rotator X 8-10 @ 2010 rest 45s X 3 sets	**Sand Workout** Dynamic Warm Up in **Sand** **A:** 2 Legged Bounding in Sand X 4 reps rest 60s 6 sets **B1:** Overhead Goal Vertical Jump X 3 rest 60s X 5 sets **C:** 30 yd agility slalom run (cones 5-8 yards apart) in the sand X 6 sets 60-120s rest between sets **D:** 5-10-20 yd shuttle sprint X 5 sets 60-120 rest between sets **E:** 80's on turf X 6 sets 45s rest between sets	

Then there is two-a-day training.......

"In 2007, researchers compared the effects of one a day and twice-a-day training in ten nationally ranked competitive weightlifters. After the three week study period, the two a day training group had twice the gain in EMG muscle activation results, as well as much more favorable increases in testosterone and testosterone/cortisol ratios (12).

Many national teams have taken the two a day approach with great success by combining several short duration, high intensity workouts throughout the day. The shorter workouts allow the body to keep cortisol levels at bay while keeping testosterone optimal. Multiple workouts also allow the athletes to train and eat without gaining excessive bodyfat due to the positive glucose tolerance, improved insulin sensitivity, and the aforementioned increases in testosterone to cortisol ratios.

On an acute level, the effects of twice-a-day training can be just as important as the long-term effects. Research out of Finland tested those effects. After two high intensity training sessions in one day, the researchers studied various strength, EMG, and hormonal parameters in the subjects. Though decreases in EMG and isometric strength were seen, increases in testosterone were measured during the second workout of the day, followed by a drop in these hormones post workout. The researchers concluded that acute hormonal and neuromuscular responses could be elicited with two a day high intensity training (5).

The same research team then studied the same eight weightlifters through one week of two a day training sessions, monitoring the same physiological variables. Once again, decreases in EMG and isometric strength were seen, while significant increases in free and total testosterone were seen during the second training session of each day. One of the most interesting findings of this study was the testosterone rebound that occurred. The researchers found the T levels to gradually decrease as the week went on, but after only one day of rest, the T levels had rebounded back to the baseline levels measured before the training started. If the study had been longer, with T level measurements during the rest and recovery periods, the T levels could have potentially rebounded to even greater levels. It is for this reason that phases of hard training followed by proper recovery can lead to dramatic gains in strength, power, and hypertrophy [6]. "

The beauty of two-a-day programming is that it allows for multiple capacities to be trained each week with adequate rest/days off. Examples of how sandpit training has been utilized in two-a-day programming include:

Weeks 1-4	Day 1	Day 2	Day 3	Day 4
AM Emphasis	Relative Strength Upper Body	Relative Strength Lower Body	Dynamic Effort Upper Body	Dynamic Effort Lower Body, Olympic Lift, Plyometric,
Rep Ranges:	1-5	1-5	1-5	1-5
Sets:	20-32 total sets	20-32 total sets	20-32 total sets	20-32 total sets
Tempo:	3010, 32X1, 2010	3010, 32X1, 2010	X0X0, 21X0, 20X1	X0X0, 21X0, 20X1
Rest Interval:	120-300s	120-300s	45-60s	45-75s
PM Emphasis	Upper Body Hypertrophy	Modified Strongman Tire Flips, Super Yoke on hard surface Kettlebell Throws, Farmer Carry, Overhead Goal Jumping in the sand	Upper Body Emphasis Modified Strongman Hand Over Hand Atlas Stone Push in Sand Hand Over Hand Rope Pull In Sand Overhead Slosh Stick Carry in Sand	Sprint and Agility Training in the sand or on turf
Rep Ranges	7-9, 8-10, 10-12, supersets, giant sets	N, Distance, Time, 1-5 reps	N, Distance, Time, 1-5 reps	Autoregulatory, N
Sets	20-32 total sets	<60min	<60min	N
Tempo	4020, 3030	NA, Explosive	NA	NA
Rest Interval	45-60s	60-240s	60-240s	N

As can be seen, sandpit training can be added to many periodization models, either on off-days from lifting or as a second workout with two-a-day training. When combined with proper weight training, modified strongman work, and field work, sandpit training can have a dramatic effect on speed, agility, conditioning, caloric expenditure, and more.

Examples of conventional and unconventional sandpit workouts:

Sample Speed and Agility Sandpit Workout 1

Exercise	Reps	Sets	Tempo	Rest Interval
A1: Overhead Kettlebell Throws	3-5	6	X0X0	30s
A2: Overhead Goal Counter Movement Jumps in the sand	2-3	6	NA	120s
B1: High Hurdle Hops in the Sand	3-5	5	NA	45s
B2: 30 yd 5 cone agility sprint in sand	30yds	5	NA	90s
C1: Hand Over Hand Atlas Stone Push Slalom	30 yds.	4	NA	15s
C2: Heavy Bag Carry In the sand	30 yds.	4	NA	90-120s
D1: 5-10-20 yd shuttle sprint	70yds total	5	NA	60s

Sample Speed and Agility Sandpit Workout 2

Exercise	Reps	Sets	Tempo	Rest Interval
A1: Agility Ladder Drills	2 per drill	6-10 sets total using 3-5 different drills	NA	45s
B1: Standing Triple Jump in the sand	1	6	NA	60s
C1: Illinois Drill in the sand		5	NA	60s
D1: Box Drill in the sand		4	NA	60s
E: Farmer Carry Slalom in the sand	30yds	6	NA	0s
E2: Overhead Slosh Stick Carry in the sand	20 yds.	6	NA	90-120s

Sample Speed and Agility Sandpit Workout 3

Exercise	Reps	Sets	Tempo	Rest Interval
A1: Agility Ladder Drills in the sand	2 per drill	6-10 total sets (3-5 drills)	NA	60s
B1: Overhead Kettlebell Throws	3	5	NA	30s
B2: Overhead Goal Countermovement Vertical Jump in the sand	2	5	NA	90-120s
C1: Chest Pass Med Ball Throw to 10 yd sprint in the sand	3	5	NA	60s
D1: Low Hurdle Jumps in the sand	5	5	NA	30s
D2: 4 cone slalom agility sprint in the sand	20 yds.	5	NA	60s
E: Hand Over Hand Rope Pull	20yds	5	NA	0s
E2: 2 Hand Atlas Stone Ball Push	20 yds.	5	NA	90-120s

Sample Speed and Agility Sandpit Workout 4

Exercise	Reps	Sets	Tempo	Rest Interval
A1: High Skips in the sand	20 yds.	6	NA	0s
A2: Backpedal Sprint in the sand	20 yds.	6	NA	45s
B1: Depth Drop in the sand	1	5	NA	45-60s
C1: Back Squat	3	5	20X0	30s
C2: 40 start position sand to hard surface 20 yd. sprint (5 yard sand 15 yd. hard surface)	1	5	NA	90-120s
D1: Forward Underhand Kettlebell Throw	3	5	NA	30s
D2: 2 Legged Bounding	3	5	NA	90-120s
E: Counter step Overhead Goal Vertical Jump in the sand	3	5	NA	30s
E2: 4 cone slalom agility sprint in the sand	20 yds.	5	NA	90-120s

Sample Weight Training and Sand Training Combined

Exercise	Reps	Sets	Tempo	Rest Interval
A1: Power Cleans on Hard Surface	2 -3	6	X0X0	30s
A2: Depth Drop (stick landing for 3 seconds) to Countermovement Vertical Jump	1	6	6	120-180s
B1: Front Squat on Hard Surface	3	5	20X0	30s
B2: 10 yard sprint on Sand	10 yds.	5	NA	90-120s
C1: Forward Underhand Kettlebell Throws	3	5	NA	30s
C2: Broad Jump	1	5	NA	60-90s
D1: 30 yard Slalom Agility Sprint	30yds	4	NA	60s
E: Hand Over Hand Atlas Stone Push	20yds	3	NA	0s
E2: Hand Over Hand Atlas Stone Pull	20 yds.	3	NA	90-120s

Sample General Preparation Sandpit Workout

Exercise	Reps	Sets	Tempo	Rest Interval
A1: Med Ball Chest Pass throw **A2:** Broad Jump In Sand	3-5 2-3	6 6	X0X0 NA	30s 120s
B1: Lateral Hurdle Hops in the Sand	3-5/leg	5	NA	45s
C1: Bounding in the sand	20 yds.	4	NA	15s
D1: Low Crawl in the sand **D2:** Keg Carry in sand	20 yds. 40 yds.	5 5	NA NA	0s 90-120s
E: Wheelbarrow load and backward pull 20 yds.	8	1	NA	0s

Sample Conditioning Workout

Exercise	Reps	Sets	Tempo	Rest Interval
A1: Low Hurdle Jumps in the sand then zig zag sprint back through the hurdles	5	6	NA	45s
B1: 6 Cone Slalom Agility Sprint in the sand	1	6	NA	0s
B2: 30 yd sprint in the sand	1	6	NA	60s
C1: Hand Over Hand Atlas Stone Slalom Push in the sand	30 Yds.	4	NA	0s
C2: Farmer Carry Slalom in the sand	30 Yds.	4	NA	120-180s
D1: Wheelbarrow load and backward pull	2 (20yds apart)	3	NA	30s
D2: Prowler Push on hard surface	30 yds.	3	NA	120-180s

Challenge Workout 1

Exercise	Reps	Sets	Tempo	Rest Interval
A1: Burpees	1↘10 (first set 1 rep, next set 2, and so on until you complete 10 burpees)	Try to finish workout as fast as you can	NA	0s
A2: 30 yd sprint in the sand	1		NA	0s
A3: Pull-Ups	1↘10 (first set 1 rep, next set 2, and so on until you complete 10 burpees)		NA	0s
A4: Bear Crawl in the sand	1		NA	0s

Challenge Workout 2
Wheelbarrow Challenge

Exercise	Reps	Sets	Tempo	Rest Interval
A1: 2 sand piles 20 yds. apart in the sand pit. Load wheelbarrow as fast as you can. Pull it backward to the other pile. Dump and load again	Complete 20 wheel barrow load and backward pulls (down and back 10X) as fast as you can.	1	NA	0s Try to complete in under 20 minutes

Challenge Workout 3
Clean to 15yd Sand Shuttle Sprint

Exercise	Reps	Sets	Tempo	Rest Interval
A1: Power Clean	1➘5 (first set 5 rep, next set 4, and so on until you get to 1 rep)		X0X0	0s
A2: 15 yd shuttle sprint in the sand	3 down and backs after each set of cleans		NA	0s Try to complete in under 5-6 minutes

Challenge Workout 4
Sand Bag Shuttle

Exercise	Reps	Sets	Tempo	Rest Interval
A1: Stack 10 sand bags in two separate piles. Set a marker 10 yards away. Grab a sand bag and sprint it to the marker. Sprint back and grab the next bag and so on. Then sprint them all back to start one at a time. Complete as fast as you can.	1	3	NA	180-240s

Challenge Workout 5
Atlas Stone Hand Over Hand Push/Pull Medley

Exercise	Reps	Sets	Tempo	Rest Interval
A1: Start with 5 atlas stones (heavier to lighter) on a line. Hand over hand push or pull each stone 20 yards starting with the heaviest stone first. Try to complete all five stones as fast as you can.	1	3	NA	180-240s

Challenge Workout 6
Obstacle Course

Exercise	Reps	Sets	Tempo	Rest Interval
A1: Over Under Hurdle 10 Hurdles **A2:** 10 Cone slalom agility sprint (50 yds. total) **A3:** 25 yd low crawl A4: Heavy Bag Carry X 25 yds. **A5:** Hand over hand rope pull X 25 yds. **A6:** Hand Over Hand Atlas Stone Push X 25 yds.		3-5		180s Try to complete in under 3 minutes

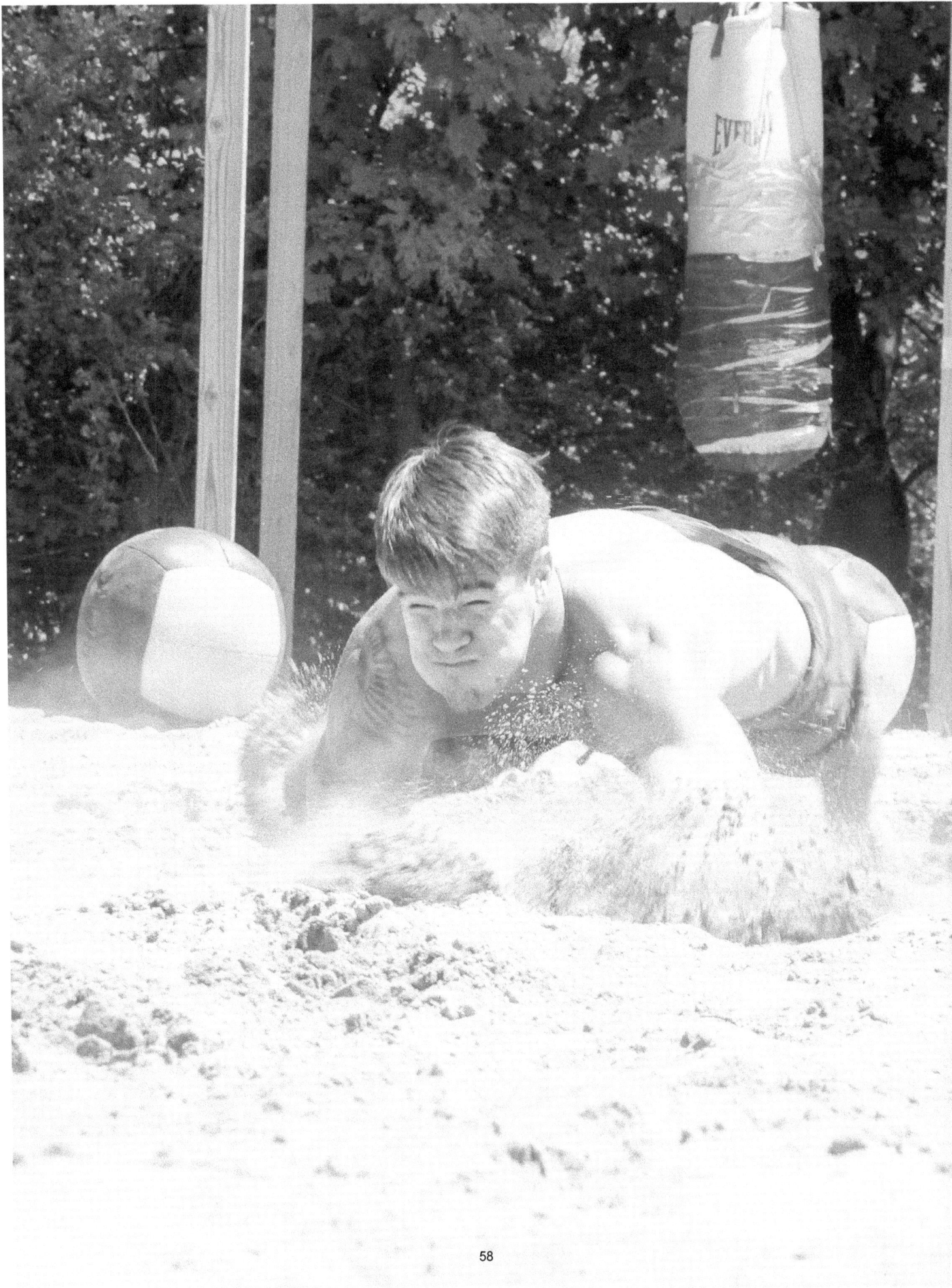

Chapter IV

Sand Training Exercise Library

2 Feet In High Knees Agility Ladder Drill In Sand

Classification: Warm Up/Quickness

Exercise Prerequisites: Avoid if chronic neck, knee, shoulder or low back pain.

Movement: Set up an agility ladder in the sand. Start facing one end of the agility ladder. Perform high knees with either one foot per rung or both feet per rung. Minimize ground contact time by trying to keep the heels off the sand. Focus on proper arm swing mechanics and keeping the torso rigid.

Keys to Movement:
1. One or two feet per rung.
2. Minimize ground contact time.
3. Maintain proper arm swing mechanics and keep the torso rigid.

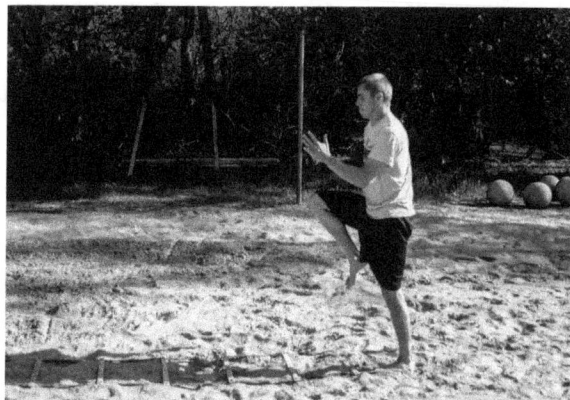

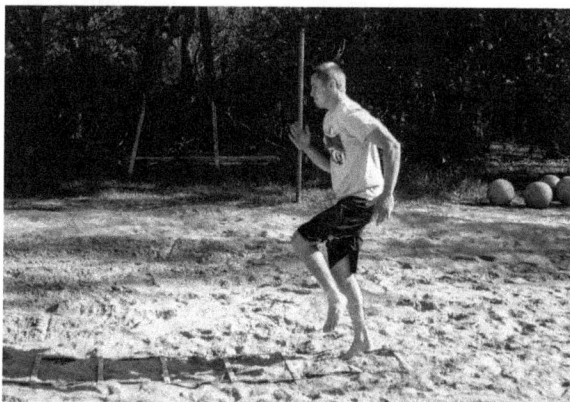

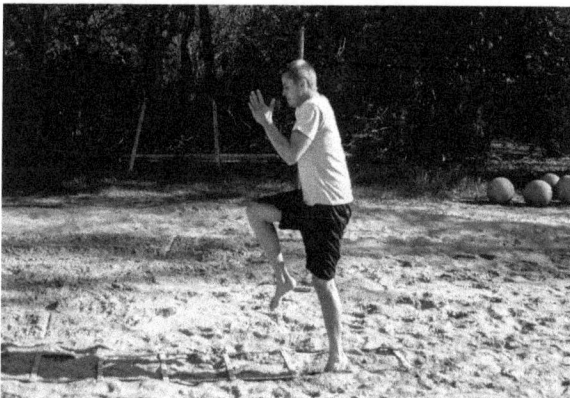

2 Legged Bounding In the Sand

Classification: Acceleration/Speed/Movement Quality

Exercise Prerequisites: Avoid if chronic neck, knee, shoulder or low back pain.

Movement: Broad jump out. As soon as you land, minimize contact time and perform again for pre-determined reps or distance.

Keys to Movement:
1. Try to cover as much distance as possible per jump utilizing optimal broad jump technique.
2. Keep the torso rigid and minimize ground contact times.

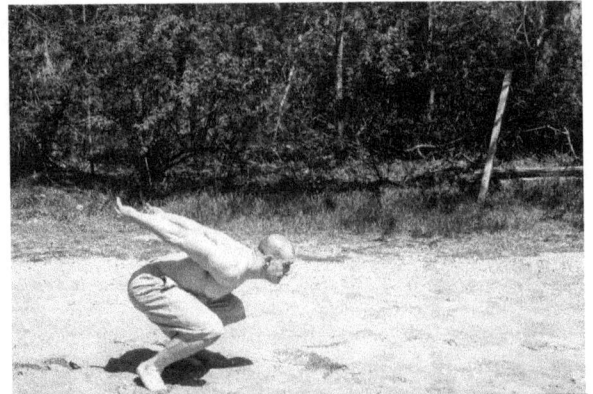

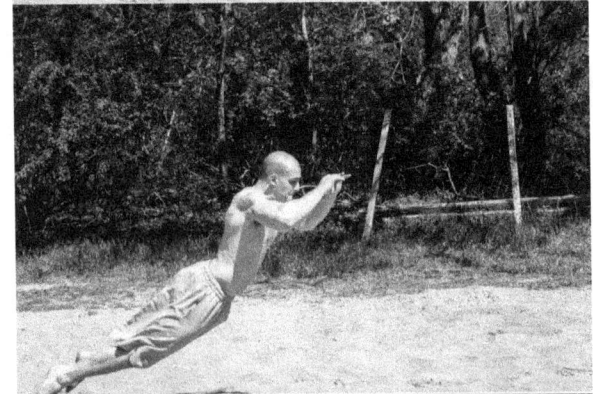

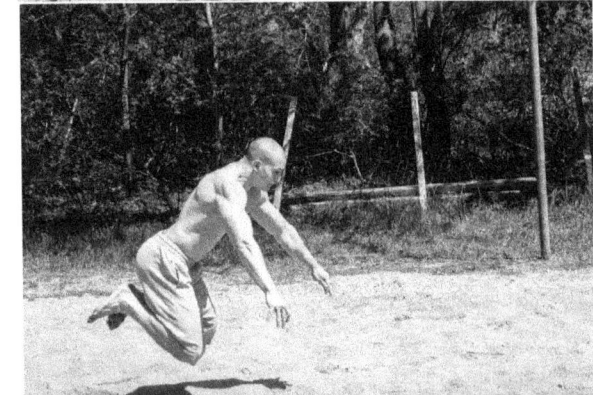

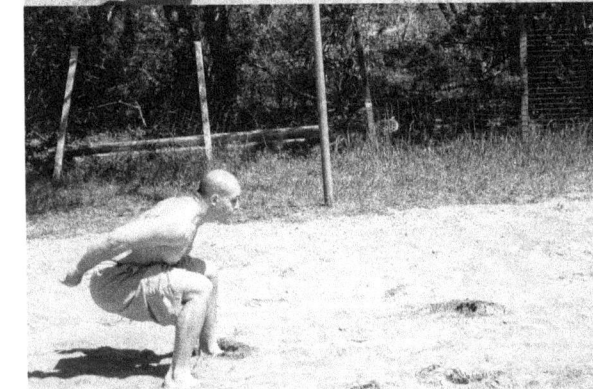

5-10-5 Pro Agility In The Sand

Classification: Agility

Exercise Prerequisites: Avoid if chronic neck, knee, shoulder or low back pain.

Movement: Set up three lines or markers, one at baseline, one 5 yards out, and one 10 yards out. Begin at the 5 yard marker standing sideways to the direction you will be sprinting. Accelerate to the 10 yard marker touching the line with your hands. Rapidly change direction and accelerate to the baseline marker and touch with your hand. Rapidly change direction and accelerate back through the initial start line (in this case the 5 yard marker).

Keys to Movement:

1. Start at the 5 yard marker standing sideways to the direction you will be sprinting.
2. Accelerate to the 10 yard marker, rapidly change direction and accelerate to the baseline. Once again rapidly change direction and accelerate through the start line.

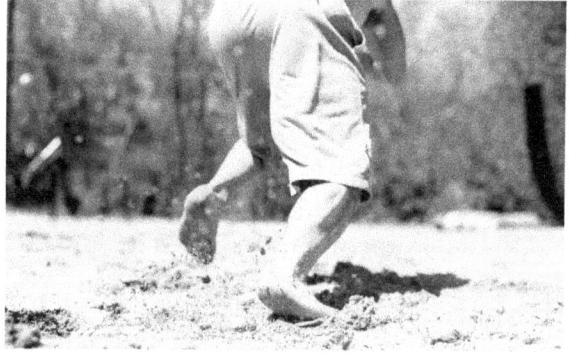

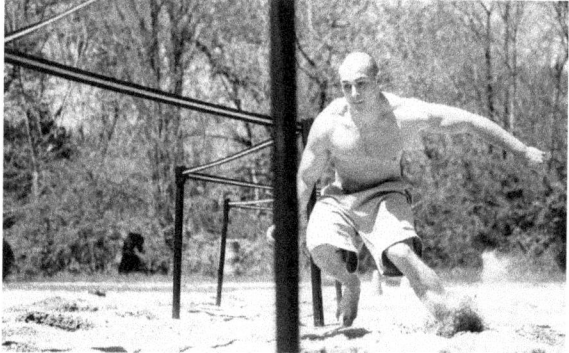

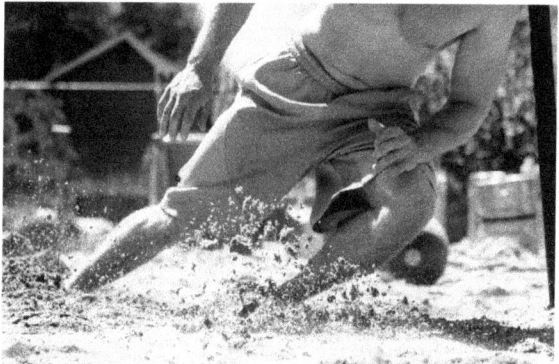

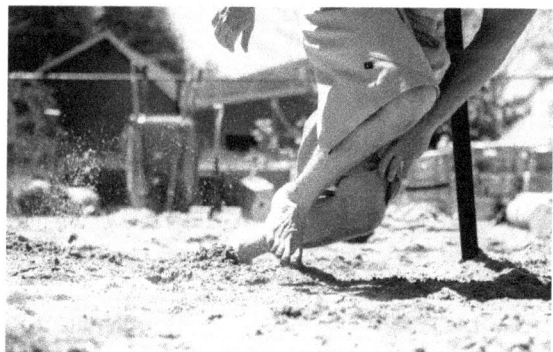

5 to 20 Yard Acceleration In The Sand From 40 or Track Start Position

Classification: Speed/Acceleration

Exercise Prerequisites: Avoid if chronic neck, knee, shoulder or low back pain.

Movement: Set up in a 40 yard dash or track start position. Trying to keep your eyes down on the ground in front of you and torso leaning, accelerate through the sand as fast as you can.

Keys to Movement:
1. Start in a 40 yard dash or track start position.
2. Keep eyes looking down in front of you with torso leaning.

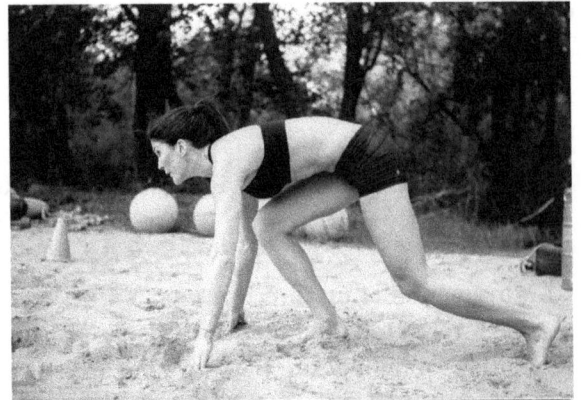

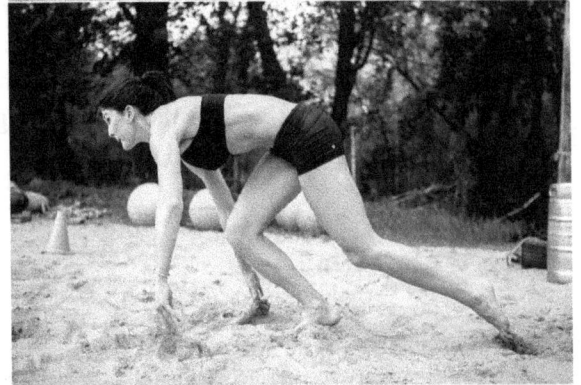

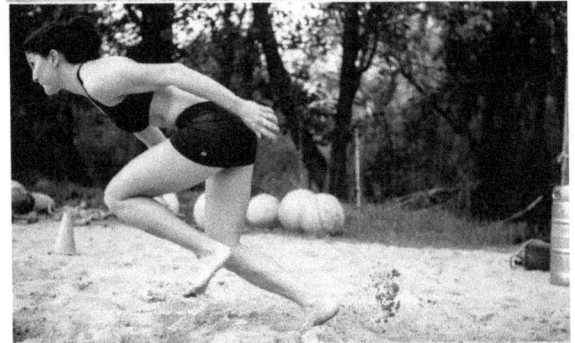

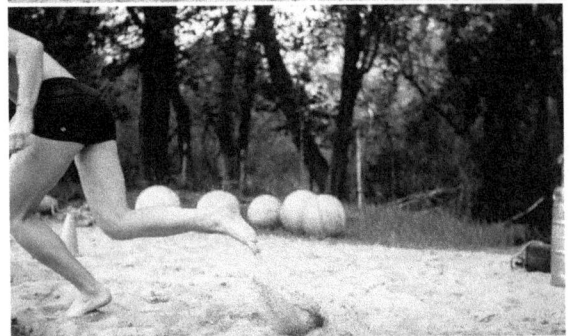

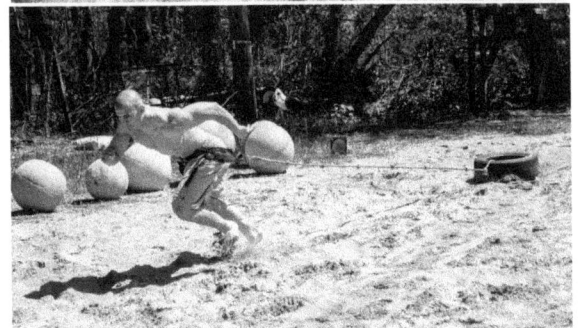

Ali Shuffle Agility Ladder Drill In The Sand

Classification: Warm Up/Quickness

Exercise Prerequisites: Avoid if chronic neck, knee, shoulder or low back pain.

Movement: Stand on the side of the agility ladder at the first rung. Jump slightly and scissor kick legs so that one foot lands in the ladder and one lands behind you outside of the ladder. Continue this motion down the ladder, switching legs as you travel to each rung.

Keys to Movement:
1. Minimize heel contact and ground contact time.
2. Keep hips and shoulders squared to the ladder.
3. Maintain stable torso.

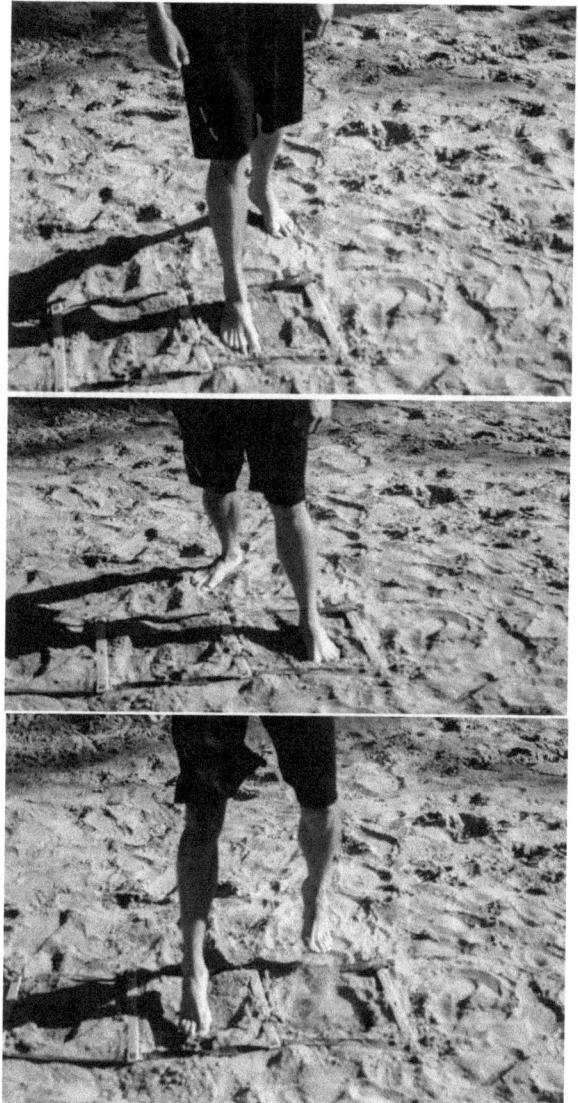

Atlas Stone Lift And Chest Press Throw

Classification: Total Body

Exercise Prerequisites: Avoid if chronic neck, knee, shoulder or low back pain.

Movement: Start with feet wider than hips and atlas stone between to slightly in front of your feet. Depending on the size of the stone, back health, experience, etc. utilize your optimal lifting posture. Some athletes prefer lordotic posture with smaller stones while others are more comfortable using a kyphotic/rounded posture for lifting the stones. Once you have lifted the stone to top of thigh/hip height cradle position, re-grip the stone with elbows higher than wrists. Pop your hips and roll the stone up your torso until it reaches top of chest to clavicle height. At this position, immediately change grip, catch the stone, and descend into slight dip (similar to dip in push press/jerk). From here immediately change direction, extending at the knees, hips, and toes, and press throw the stone as far out in front of you as you can.

Keys to Movement:

1. Lift the atlas stone with your preferred or optimal lifting mechanics.
2. Pop the stone up to shoulder/clavicle height.
3. Catch the stone, dip, immediately reverse direction and extend, press throwing the stone in front of you.

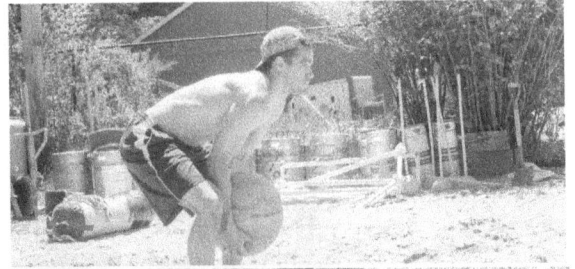

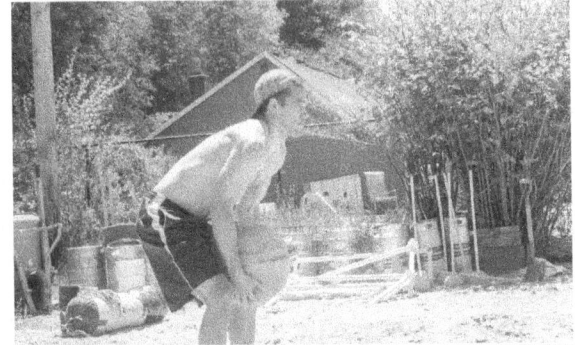

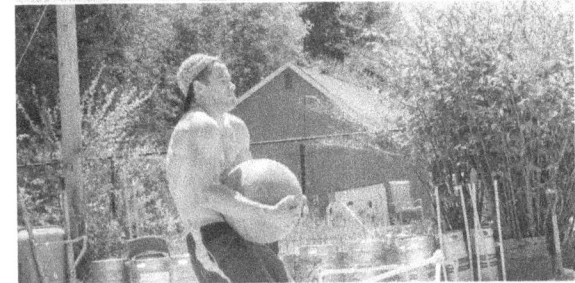

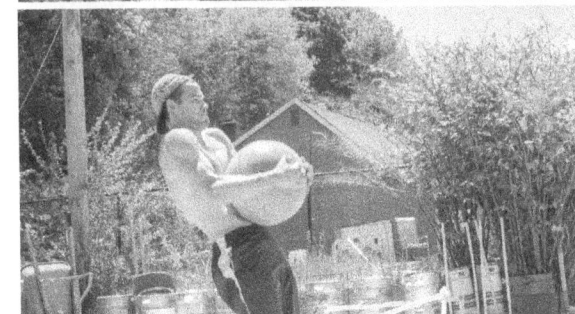

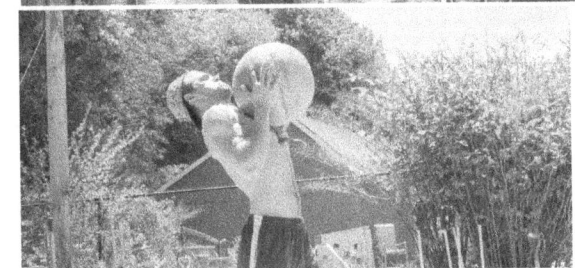

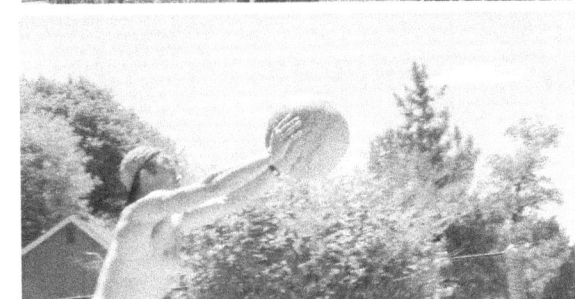

Back Squat to Broad Jump in the Sand Complex

Classification: Lower Body Strength and Power

Exercise Prerequisites: Avoid if chronic neck, knee, shoulder or low back pain.

Movement: Perform a conventional deep back squat on a solid platform near the sandpit. Rest roughly 30 seconds and perform a broad jump in the sand.

Keys to Movement:

1. Upon completion of predetermined repetitions of back squat, rest roughly 30 seconds and perform a broad jump in the sand.
2. Feel free to use accommodated resistance in the form of Bands or Chains to add to the intensity of your squats.

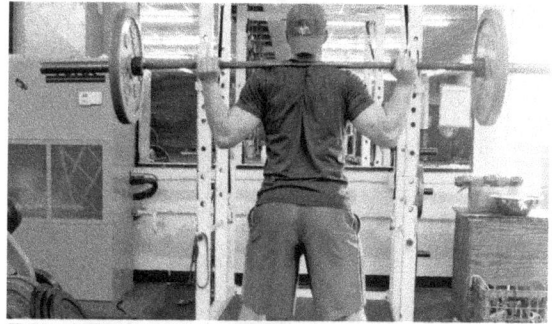

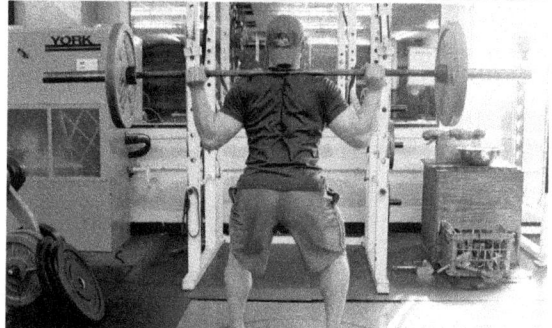

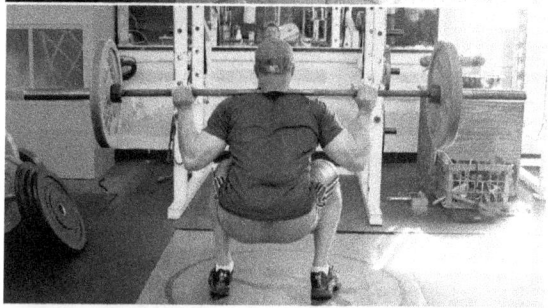

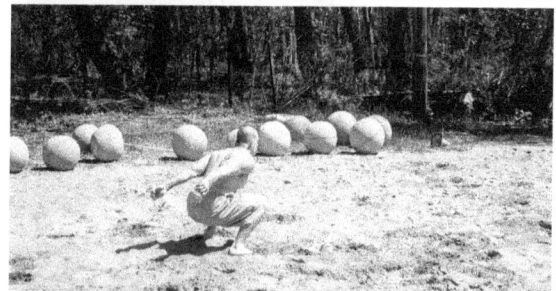

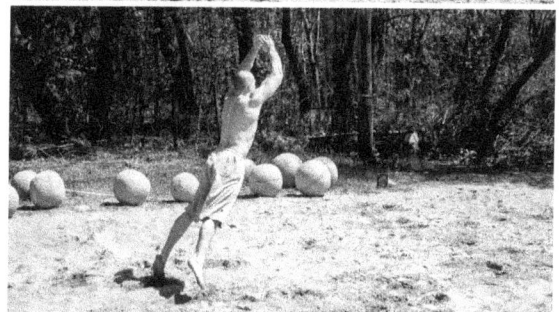

Back Squat to Depth Jump in the Sand Complex

Classification: Lower Body Strength and Power

Exercise Prerequisites: Avoid if chronic neck, knee, shoulder or low back pain.

Movement: Perform a conventional deep back squat on a solid platform near the sandpit. Rest roughly 30 seconds and perform a non-true plyometric depth jump in the sand.

Keys to movement:

1. Upon completion of predetermined repetitions of back squat, rest roughly 30 seconds and perform a non-true plyometric jump in the sand.
2. Feel free to use accommodated resistance in the form of Bands or Chains to add to the intensity of your squats.

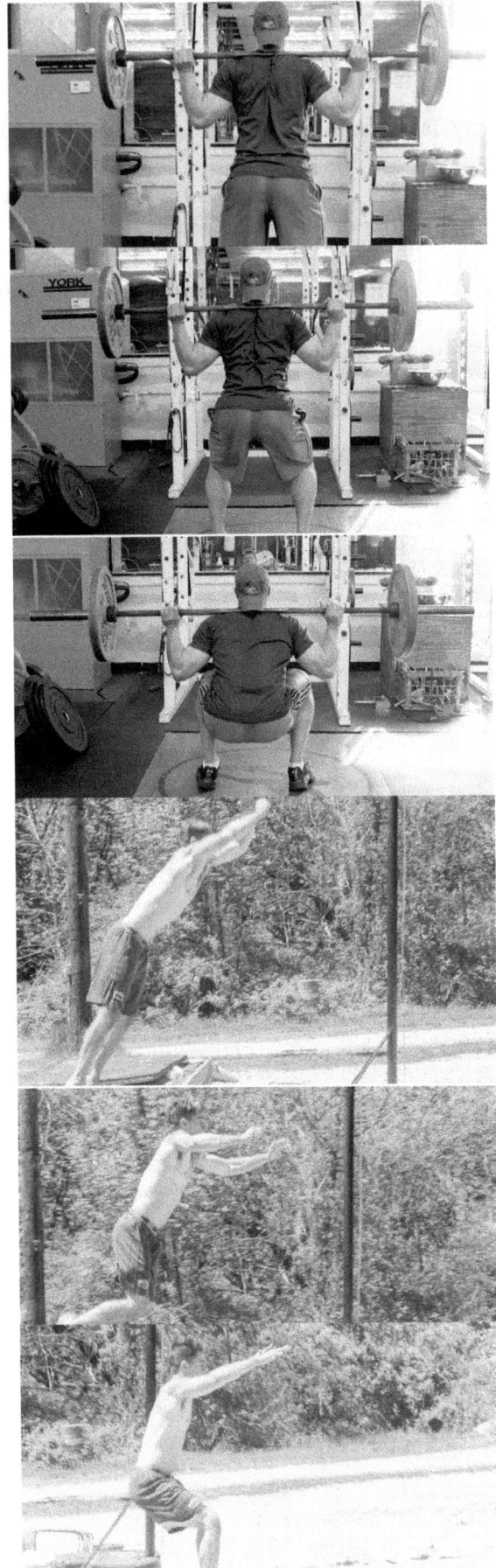

Back Squat to Chest Pass Throw in the Sand Complex

Classification: Lower Body Strength and Power

Exercise Prerequisites: Avoid if chronic neck, knee, shoulder or low back pain.

Movement: Perform a conventional deep back squat on a solid platform near the sandpit. Rest roughly 30 seconds and perform a chest pass throw in the sand with med ball, kettlebell, or implement of your choice.

Keys to Movement:

1. Upon completion of predetermined repetitions of back squat, rest roughly 30 seconds and perform an overhead throw in the sand.
2. Feel free to use accommodated resistance in the form of Bands or Chains to add to the intensity of your squats.

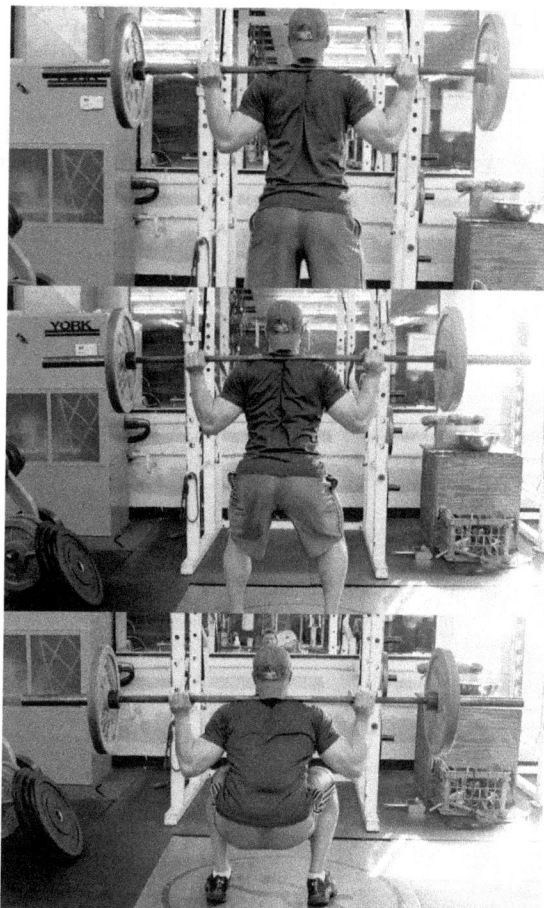

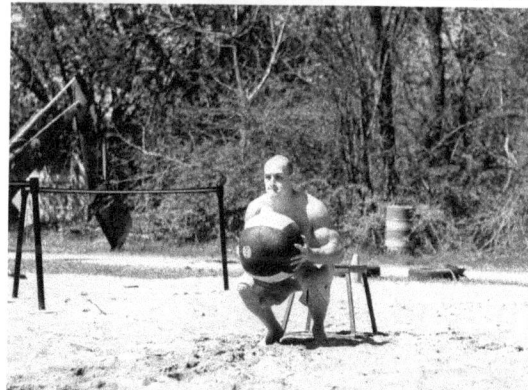

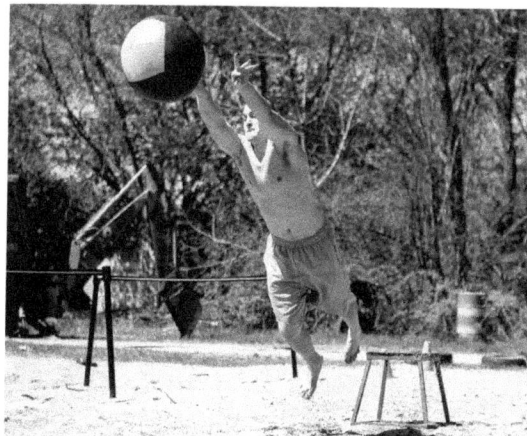

Back Squat to Resisted Sled Sprint in the Sand Complex

Classification: Lower Body Strength, Speed, and Power

Exercise Prerequisites: Avoid if chronic neck, knee, shoulder or low back pain.

Movement: Perform a conventional deep back squat on a solid platform near the sandpit. Rest roughly 30 seconds and perform a resisted sprint in the sand.

Keys to Movement:

1. Upon completion of predetermined repetitions of back squat, rest roughly 30 seconds and perform a resisted sprint in the sand.
2. Feel free to use accommodated resistance in the form of Bands or Chains to add to the intensity of your squats.

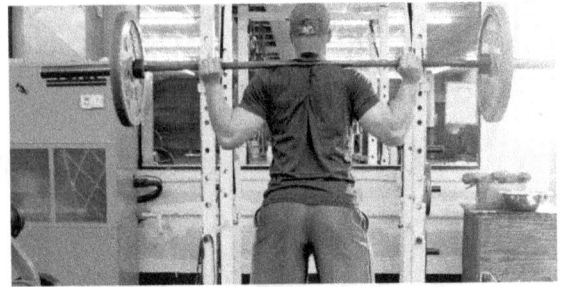

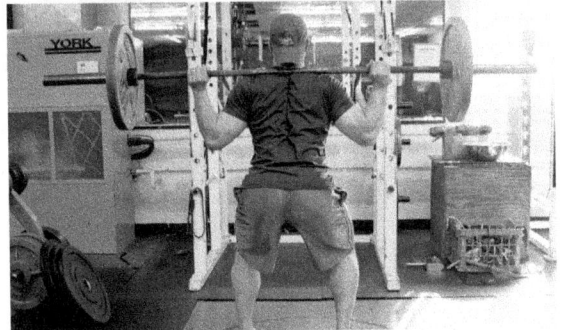

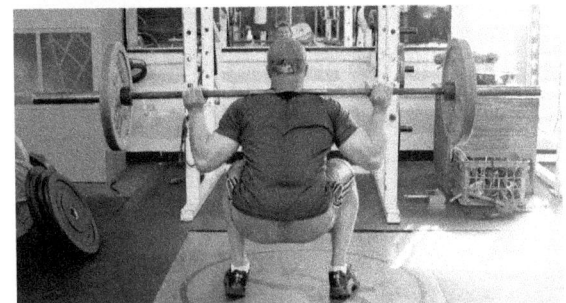

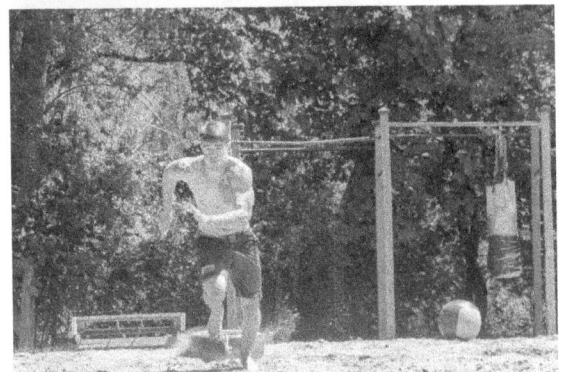

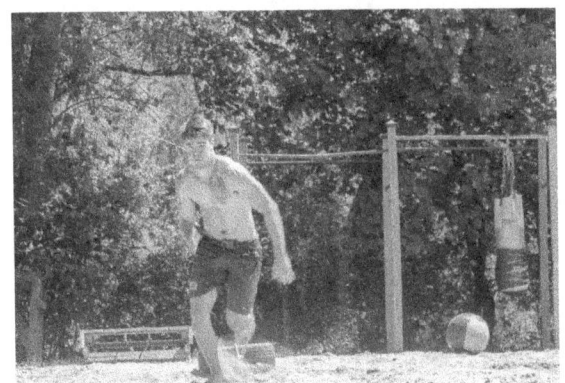

Back Squat to 15 yd. Sprint in the Sand Complex

Classification: Lower Body Strength and Speed

Exercise Prerequisites: Avoid if chronic neck, knee, shoulder or low back pain.

Movement: Perform a conventional deep back squat on a solid platform near the sandpit. Rest roughly 30 seconds and perform a short sprint in the sand.

Keys to movement:

1. Upon completion of predetermined repetitions of back squat, rest roughly 30 seconds and perform a short sprint in the sand.
2. Feel free to use accommodated resistance in the form of Bands or Chains to add to the intensity of your squats

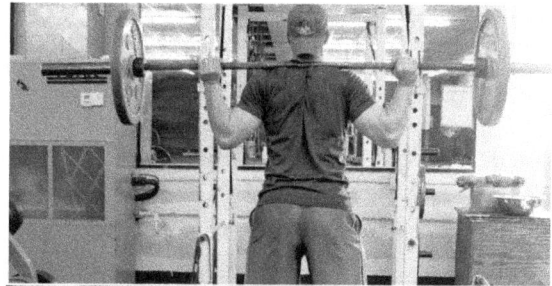

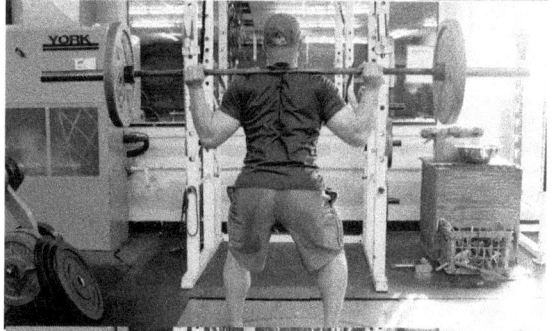

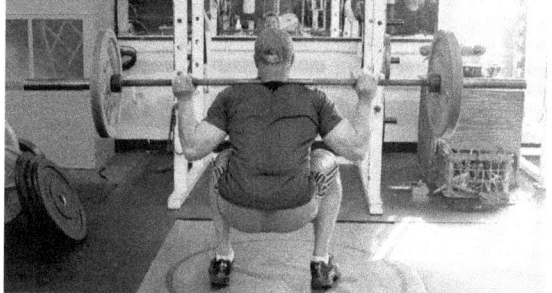

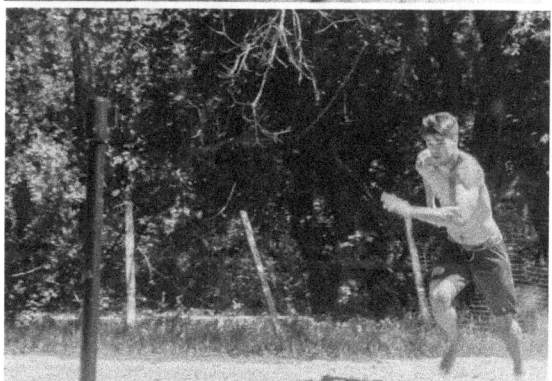

Back Squat to Vertical Jump in the Sand Complex

Classification: Lower Body Strength and Total Body Power

Exercise Prerequisites: Avoid if chronic neck, knee, shoulder or low back pain.

Movement: Perform a conventional deep back squat on a solid platform near the sandpit. Rest roughly 30 seconds and perform a vertical jump in the sand.

Keys to the Movement:

1. Upon completion of predetermined repetitions of back squat, rest roughly 30 seconds and perform a vertical jump in the sand.
2. Feel free to use accommodated resistance in the form of Bands or Chains to add to the intensity of your squats.

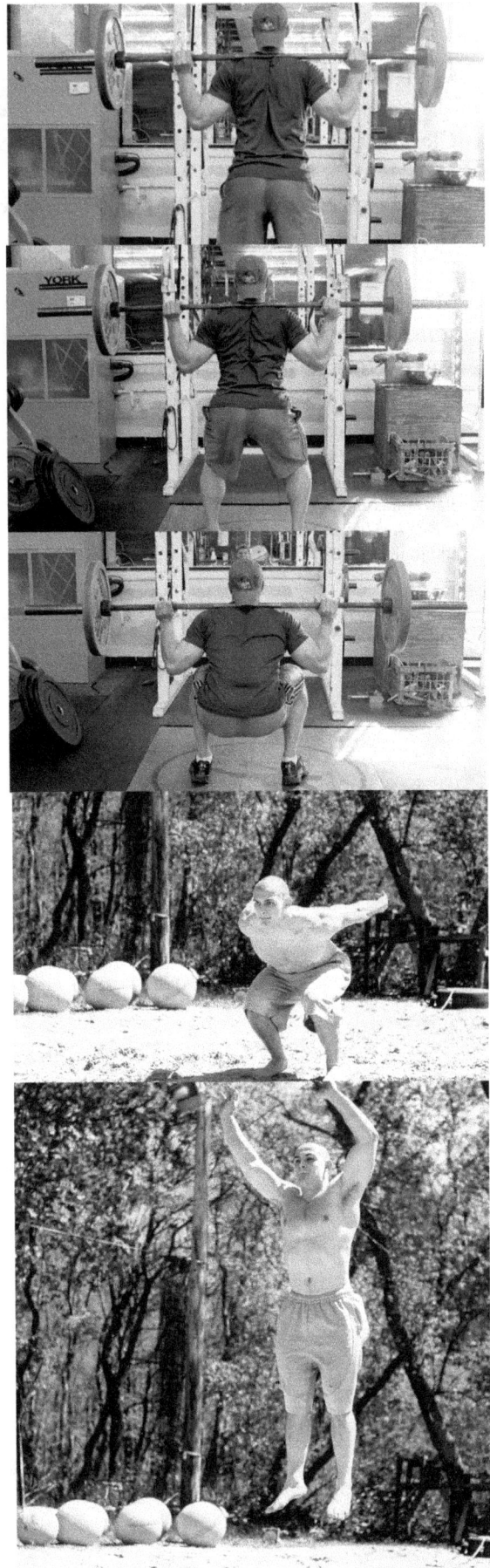

Backward Dragging in the Sand

Classification: Lower Body Strength and Conditioning

Exercise Prerequisites: Four week familiarization and adaptation to sand training is recommended prior to engaging in high intensity jump training in the sand. You may want to avoid if you have Achilles tendon, knee, hip, low back, ankle, or neck issues.

Movement: Facing a sled, heavy bag, or other dragging implement hold the rope or straps and lean back with shoulders behind hips and feet hip width apart. Keeping hips extended and shoulders behind hips begin walking backward focusing on fully extending the drive leg with each stride. Be sure not to reach back more than one foot length with the non-working leg as this can put unnecessary stress on the knee. The hips locked at 90 degrees sled drag as a viable option.

Keys to Movement:

1.   Position feet hip width apart.
2.   Lean back with hips extended and shoulders behind hips.
3.   Focus on driving through the ball of the foot.
4.   Extend the leg fully with each step.
5.   Be careful not to step too far back and this can put excessive strain on the knee.

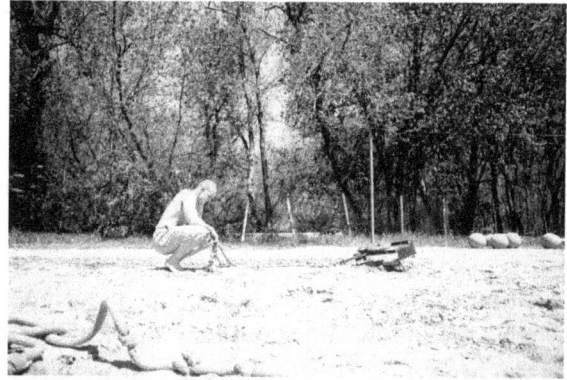

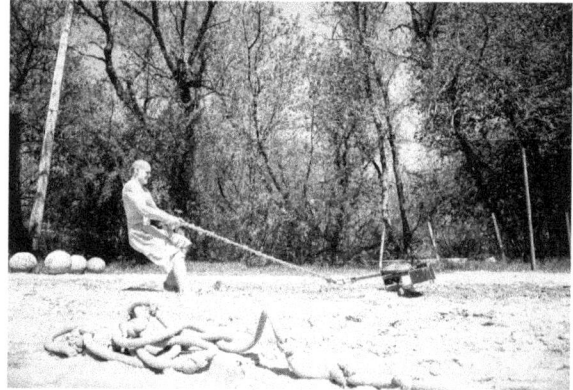

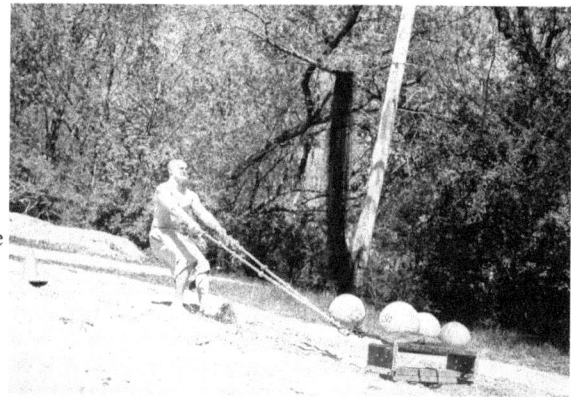

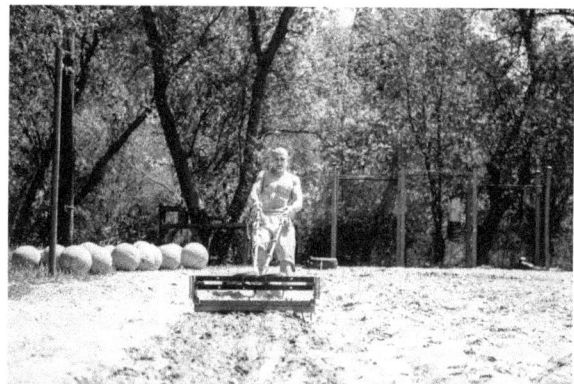

Bear Crawls in the Sand

Classification: Total Body

Exercise Prerequisites: Avoid if chronic knee, shoulder, neck or low back pain.

Movement: Start in kneeling position with hands directly below the shoulders and knees directly below the hips. Lift hips into the air so weight is distributed evenly on hands and feet. Two options for bear crawl are torso parallel to the floor or hips elevated above the shoulders. Initiate movement by stepping forward onto one hand, followed by opposite leg, etc.

Keys to Movement:
1. Start in kneeling position with hands directly below shoulders and knees directly below hips.
2. Choose either torso parallel to ground bear crawl or hips elevated above shoulder bear crawl option.

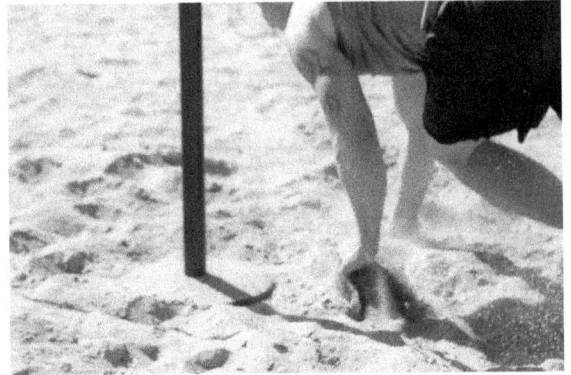

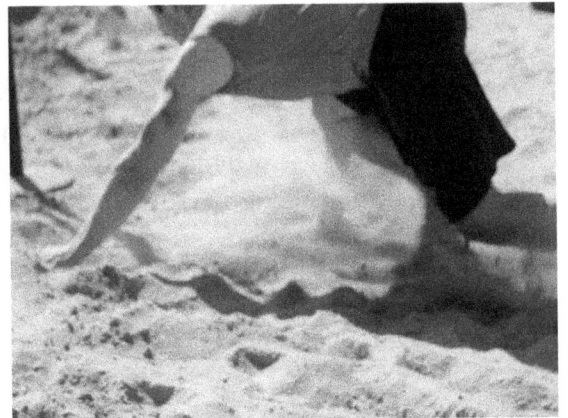

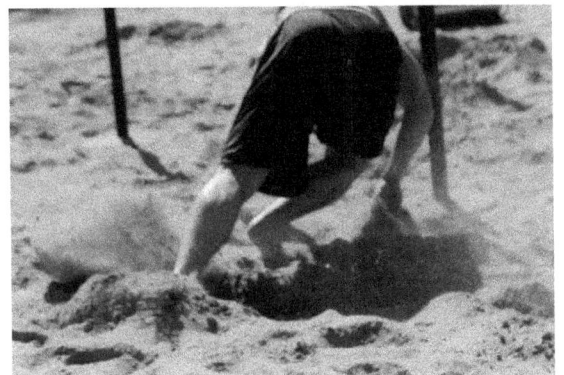

Body Squats in the Sand

Classification: Lower body

Exercise Prerequisites: Avoid if chronic knee or low back pain.

Movement: Stand with feet hip width apart or slightly wider, with toes pointing straight ahead or slightly out. Options for your hand placement include hands on your hips, behind your head, arms extended upward in the air, or arms crossed in genie position. As you begin the descent, make sure to maintain lordotic/neutral posture beginning the decent by bending your knees first (a variation is to bend at the hips first). As you sit downward, begin pushing your knees outward to ensure maximum hip muscle recruitment, while keeping the weight on the heels. Once your hamstrings touch your calves, or you have gone as low as your flexibility allows, begin to initiate the ascent. Keeping the back arched/neutral with torso rigid, focus on driving the chest up first, keeping the torso upright. Be sure to keep the heels driving into the ground, and avoid caving knees and rounding of the back.

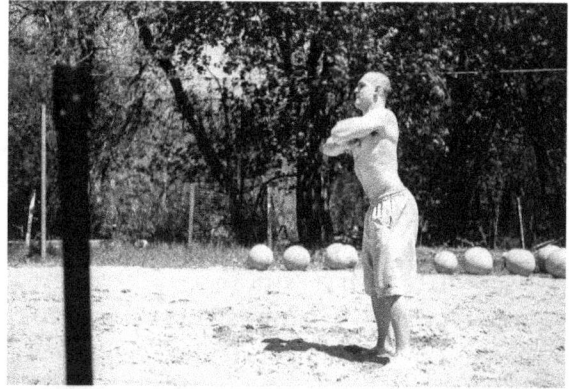

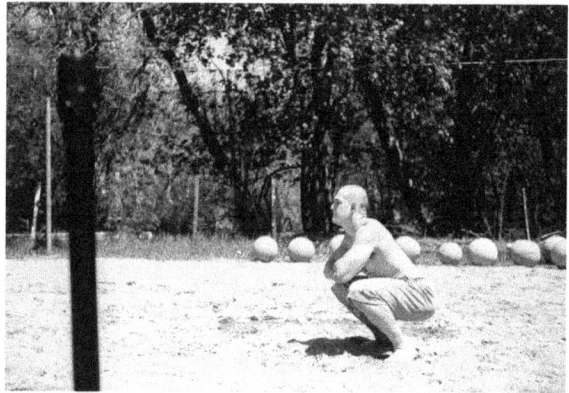

Keys to Movement:

1. Place feet hip width or slightly wider with toes pointing slightly outward.
2. Maintain neutral/lordotic posture while keeping the torso as upright as possible.
3. Bend at the knees or hips first when you begin your descent.
4. Push the knees outward, ensuring they point in the same direction as the toes throughout the movement.
5. Do not allow the heels to come off the ground or knees collapse throughout the movement.
6. Lower down until your hamstrings touch your calves or as low as your flexibility allows.
7. Initiate ascent by driving chest upward at first.

Bounding in the Sand

Classification: Speed/Acceleration/Power

Exercise Prerequisites: Avoid if chronic neck, knee, shoulder or low back pain.

Movement: Start with two to three medium running strides, then begin long strides, trying to cover as much ground as you can per stride. Focus on pulling through the sand, engaging the powerful hip extensors. Keep the torso rigid and minimize ground contact times.

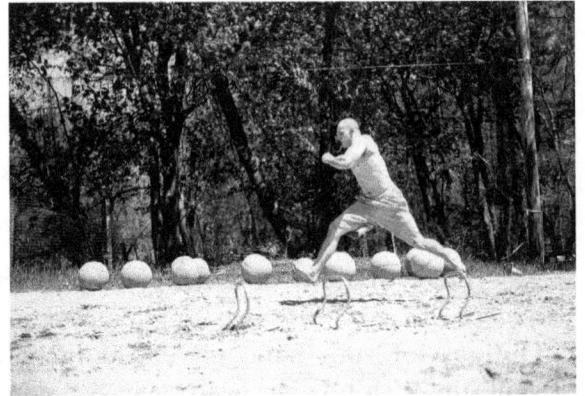

Keys to Movement:

1. Try to maximize distance covered per stride while minimizing ground contact time.
2. Keep torso rigid and focus on optimal arm swing and leg drive mechanics.

Box Drill in the Sand

Classification: Agility and Lateral Quickness

Exercise Prerequisites: Avoid if chronic neck, knee, shoulder or low back pain.

Movement: Make a box with 4 cones 10 yards apart from each other. Start at one cone. Sprint forward to the next cone. Side shuffle to the next cone. Backpedal to the next cone, and side shuffle back to start. Try to complete as fast as possible keeping a rigid upright posture throughout.

Keys to the Movement:
1. Face the same direction the entire drill.
2. Keep torso rigid throughout drill.

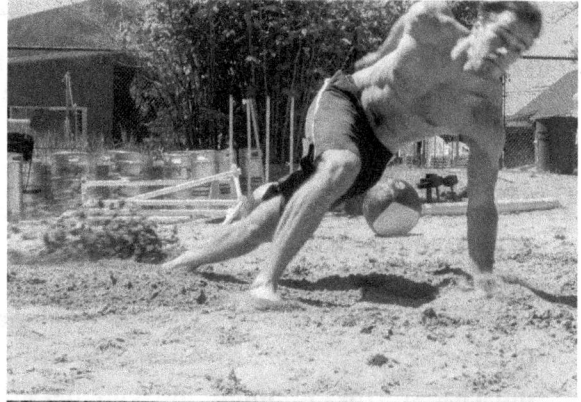

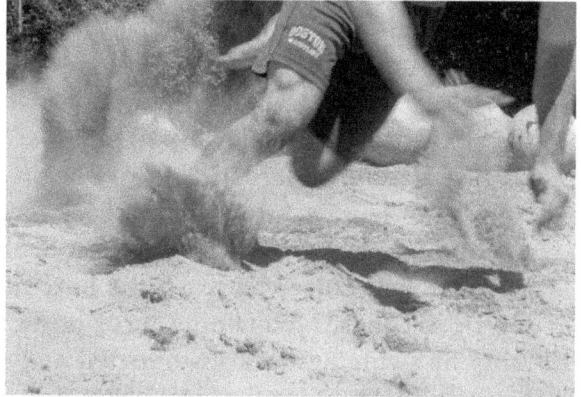

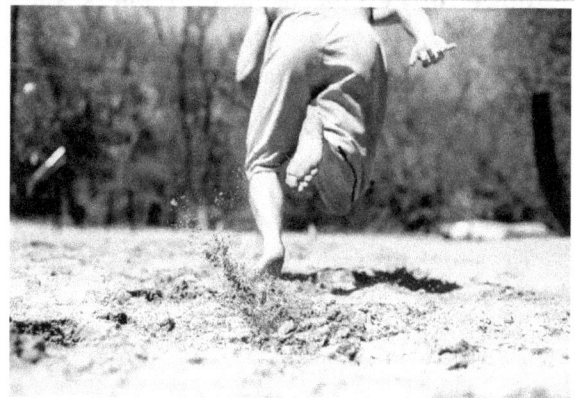

Bodyweight Box Squat Start Position to Broad Jump or Vertical Jump in the Sand

Classification: Total Body Power

Exercise Prerequisites: Avoid if chronic knee, shoulder, neck or low back pain.

Movement: This exercise is used to teach parallel squat form as well as proper activation of the glute/hamstring muscles during jumping movements. The box you choose to sit on should be a height in which when you reach the bottom of the squat, the upper thigh is parallel or slightly below parallel to the ground. Stand in front of the boxy with feet roughly hip to shoulder width apart, posture neutral to lordotic. As you begin the descent, try to maintain posture as you sit back toward the box. Keep your knees in line with your feet or slightly wider as you squat. Once you reach the box, sit on the box for 1-3 seconds. Maintaining torso posture, begin the jump by swinging the arms outward and upward, and powerfully extending the hips, knees, and ankles. Jump as high or far as possible. Stick the landing in the sand as softly as possible landing in a ¼ or ½ squat position with minimal break in torso posture.

Keys to Movement:

1. Squat down onto a box with thighs parallel to the ground at the bottom of the squat.
2. Sit on the box for 1-3 seconds.
3. Perform downward countermovement with arms and torso.
4. Rapidly change direction and jump as high or far as possible.

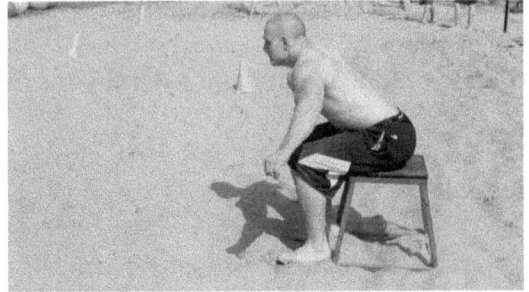

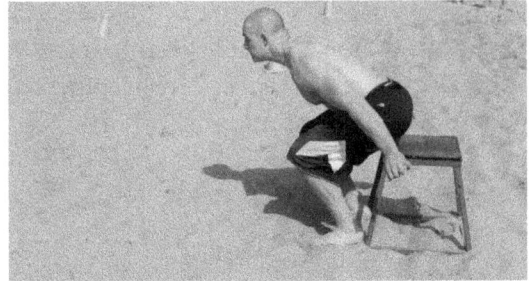

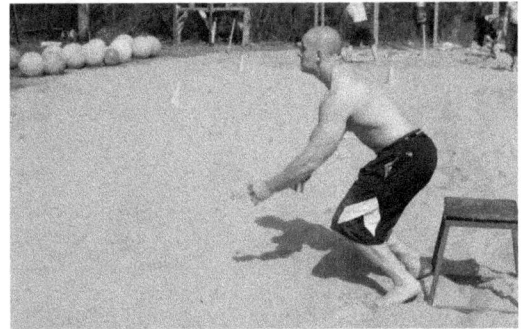

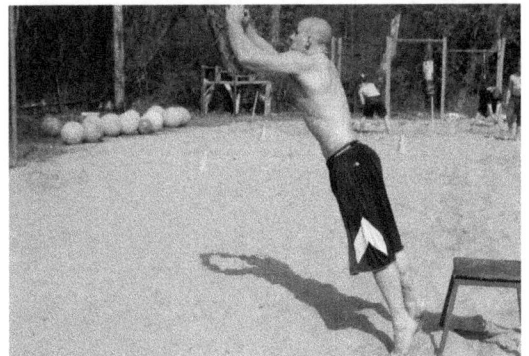

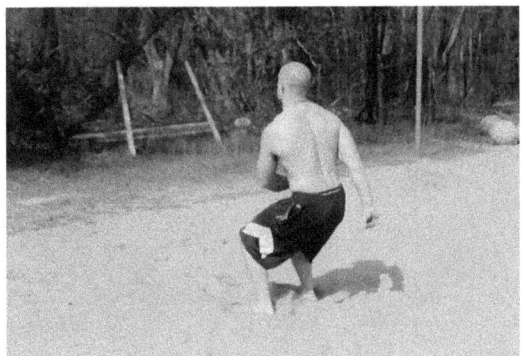

Broad Jump in the Sand

Classification: Total Body Power

Exercise Prerequisites: Four week familiarization and adaptation to sand training is recommended prior to engaging in high intensity jump training in the sand. You may want to avoid if you have Achilles tendon, knee, hip, low back, ankle, or neck issues.

Movement: The faster you perform the countermovement, the further you will jump. It is Newton's Law which states "for every action, there is an equal and opposite reaction". Picture a tennis ball bouncing against a wall. If you lightly toss the ball it may rebound 3-4 feet back to you. The reaction is equal to the action. Whereas if you throw the ball with maximal force against the wall the ball will rebound much further. For countermovement jumps, the body works in the manner.

Begin by positioning your feet roughly hip width apart, with knees and toes pointing straight ahead, and shoulders and hips squared. Swing arms directly overhead reaching as high as possible, coming on up onto your toes, with full extension in ankles, knees, spine, and shoulders. Once you have reached this extended position, swing your extended arms down as powerfully as possible, keeping your head neutral or looking forward slightly. Bend more at the hips than knees to initiate greater hamstring tension.

Once you have reached optimal glute and hamstring tension, rapidly reverse direction and swing your arms upward and outward. Powerfully extend your hips, knees, and ankles driving the body outward and upward into the air with arms reaching as out as far as possible and head looking out/upward. Try to pull your knees behind your body while in the air. Toward the end of the jump, prepare your body for landing by pulling the knees and feet back in front of the body. Land on two feet with optimal landing mechanics.

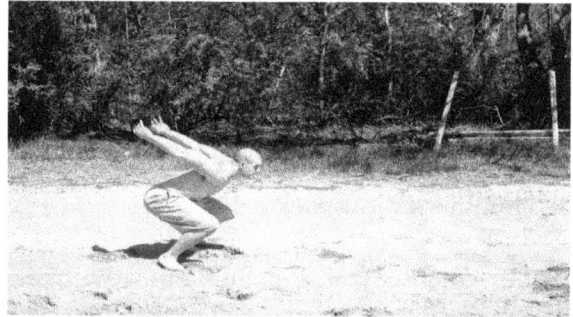

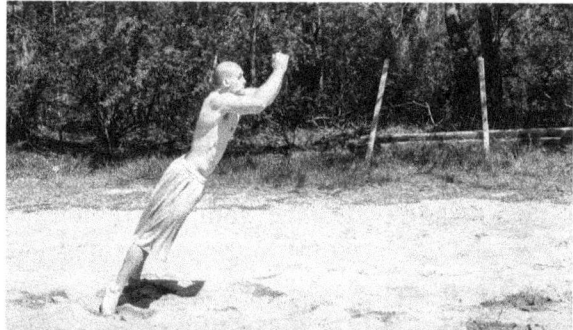

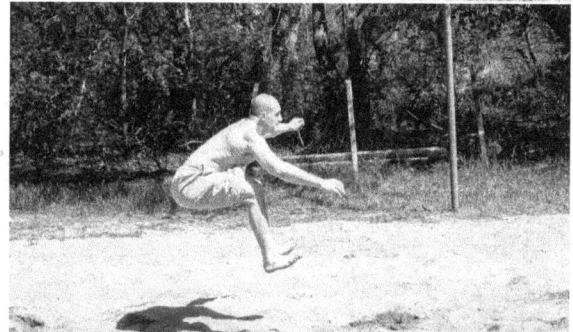

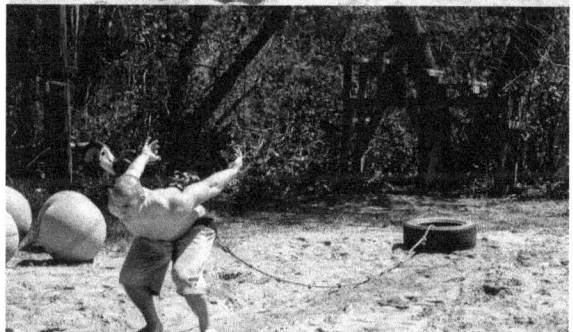

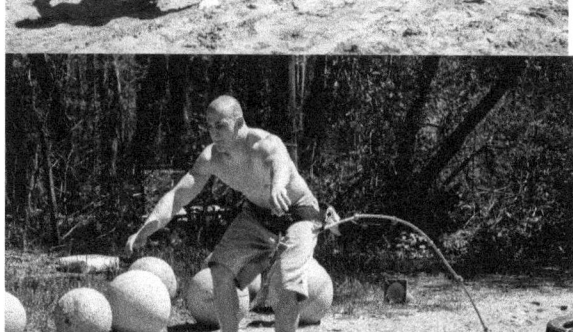

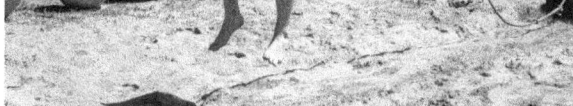

Burpee Broad Jump in the Sand

Classification: Total Body Power and/or Conditioning

Exercise Prerequisites: Avoid if chronic neck, knee, shoulder or low back pain.

Movement: Start in standing position with feet roughly hip width apart and parallel. Begin by leaning over and placing hand on the ground in front of you in push up position. Jump your feet back, keeping them together, into pushup position. Keeping angle at arm pits roughly 45 degree or less, glutes and quads contracted, descend into pushup. As you descend retract your shoulder blades and ensure that your hips do not sink toward the sand. Descend until your upper arms are parallel to the ground or lower. After you have reached your lowest desired point, begin to press the body up by driving the palms into the sand and extending the elbows. Be sure to keep hips extended, with glutes and quads contracted. At the top of the pushup, jump both feet together toward your hands, keeping hands in contact with the sand. Once your feet hit the sand jump as far as you can using a counter movement jump arm swing. Land with optimal landing mechanics and perform for desired repetitions.

Keys to Movement:

1. Start standing with feet parallel and hip width apart.
2. Drop down to technically sound pushup position by placing hands on the sand first.
3. Perform pushup then jump to your feet.
4. Once your feet come in contact with the sand, jump as far as you can, utilizing countermovement jump arm swing mechanics.
5. Try to land with optimal landing mechanics.

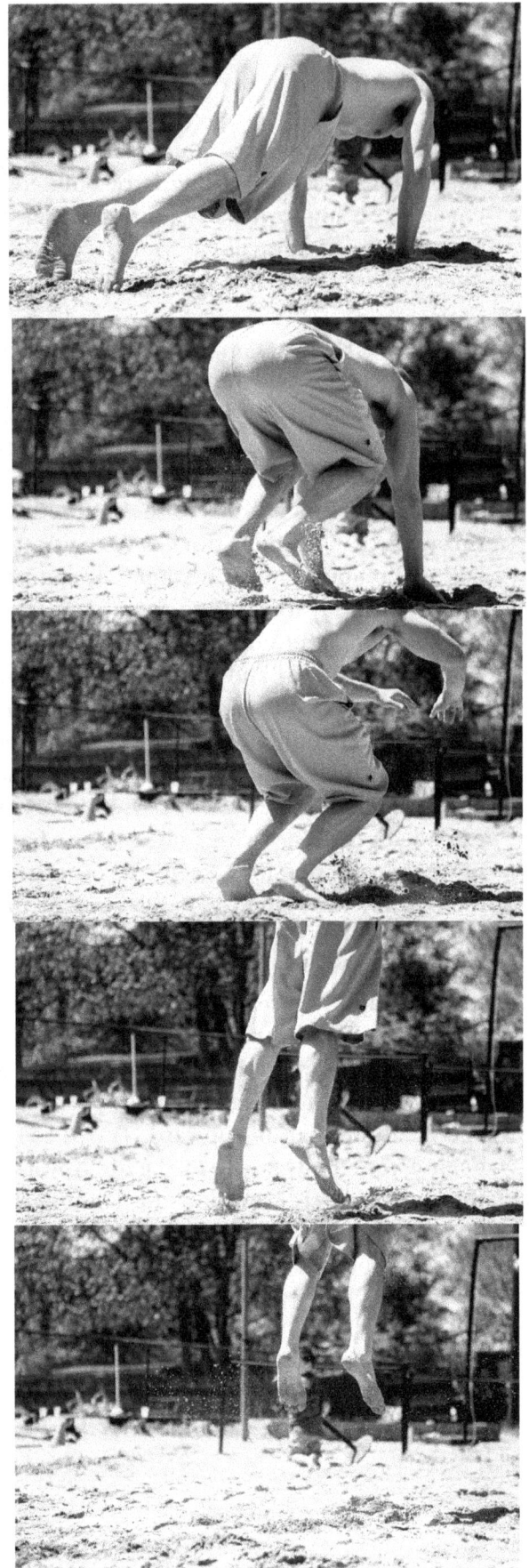

Burpee to Vertical Jump in the Sand

Classification: Total Body Power

Exercise Prerequisites: Avoid if chronic neck, knee, shoulder or low back pain.

Movement: Start in standing position with feet roughly hip width apart and parallel. Begin by leaning over and placing hand on the ground in front of you in push up position. Jump your feet back, keeping them together, into pushup position. Keeping angle at arm pits roughly 45 degree or less, glutes and quads contracted, descend into pushup. As you descend retract your shoulder blades and ensure that your hips do not sink toward the sand. Descend until your upper arms are parallel to the ground or lower. After you have reached your lowest desired point, begin to press the body up by driving the palms into the sand and extending the elbows. Be sure to keep hips extended, with glutes and quads contracted. At the top of the pushup, jump both feet together toward your hands, keeping hands in contact with the sand. Once your feet hit the sand jump as high as you can using a counter movement jump arm swing. Land with optimal landing mechanics and perform for desired repetitions.

Keys to Movement:

1. Start standing with feet parallel and hip width apart.
2. Drop down to technically sound pushup position by placing hands on the sand first.
3. Perform pushup then jump to your feet.
4. Once your feet come in contact with the sand, jump as high as you can, utilizing countermovement jump arm swing mechanics.
5. Try to land with optimal landing mechanics.

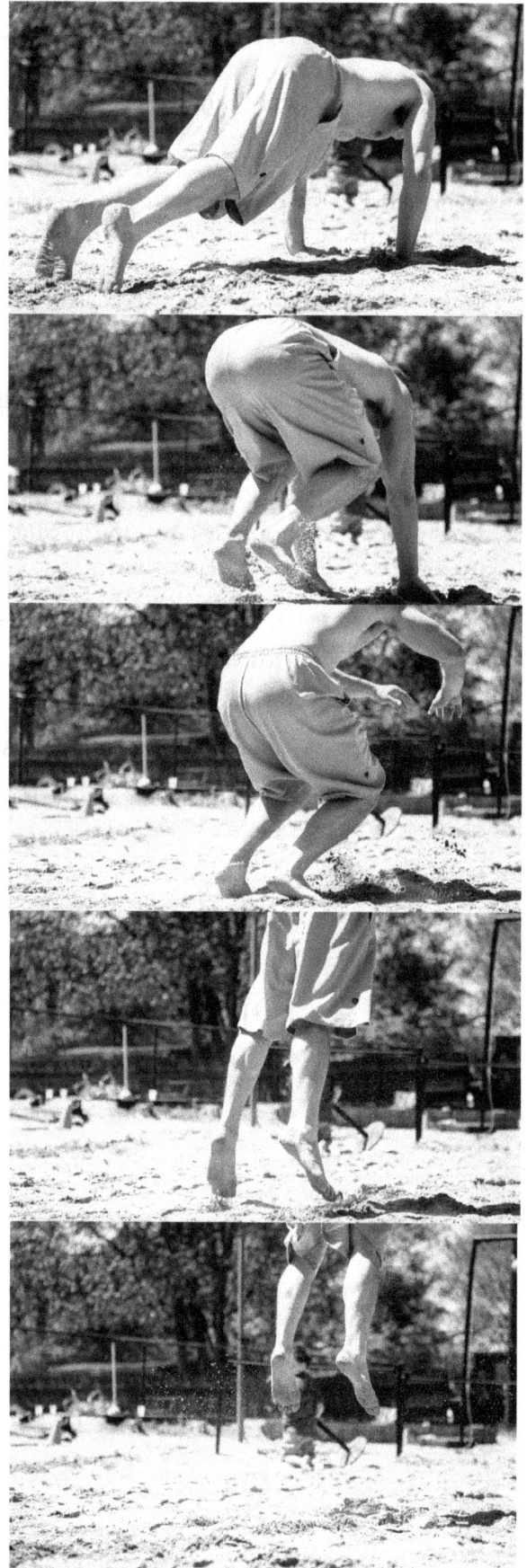

Burpee Over Unders in the Sand

Classification: Total Body Power/Conditioning

Exercise Prerequisites: Four week familiarization and adaptation to sand training is recommended prior to engaging in high intensity jump training in the sand. You may want to avoid if you have Achilles tendon, knee, hip, low back, ankle, or neck issues.

Movement: Stand sideways to a rope or long hurdle roughly knee to hip height. Jump laterally over the hurdle and drop into a burpee position. Trying to maintain same body position relative to the hurdle/rope, slide under the hurdle, jump to your feet similar to a burpee, and jump back over the hurdle. Perform for predetermined time or repetitions.

Keys to the Movement:

1. Stand sideways next to a long hurdle or rope roughly knee to hip height.
2. Laterally jump over the hurdle.
3. Drop down to pushup position and slide under the hurdle.
4. Jump to your feet and jump back over the hurdle.

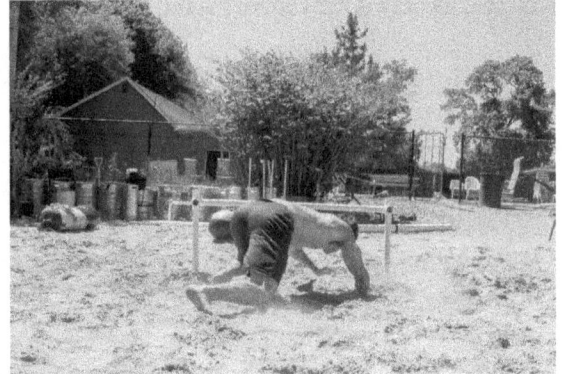

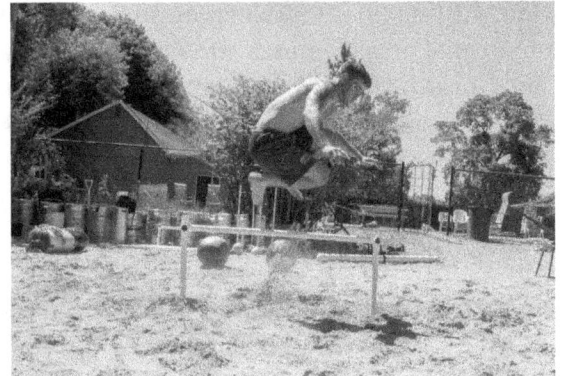

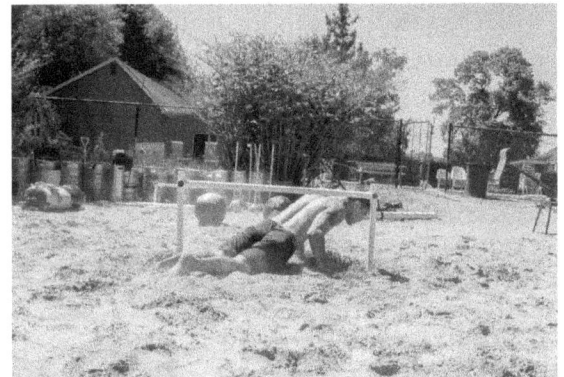

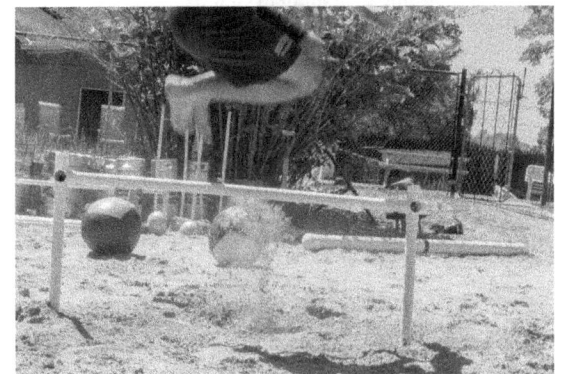

Crocodile Walk in the Sand

Classification: Core/Shoulders/Arms Strength and Conditioning

Exercise Prerequisites: Avoid if chronic knee, shoulder, neck or low back pain.

Movement: Start laying flat on the ground with hand and feet in optimal pushup position, with hands directly below shoulder. Lift body slightly by performing quarter pushup, keeping elbows tight to the body. Keeping torso rigid and parallel to the ground, begin by taking a small step with one arm, then small step with foot. Do not allow legs to bend. Alternate steps. When done properly, movement looks similar to that of crocodile crawling.

Movement Mechanics:

1. Start in quarter pushup position with upper arms and torso parallel to the sand.
2. Keeping legs straight and torso/arms parallel to the ground, take small steps alternating between hands and feet.
3. Perform for predetermined time or distance.

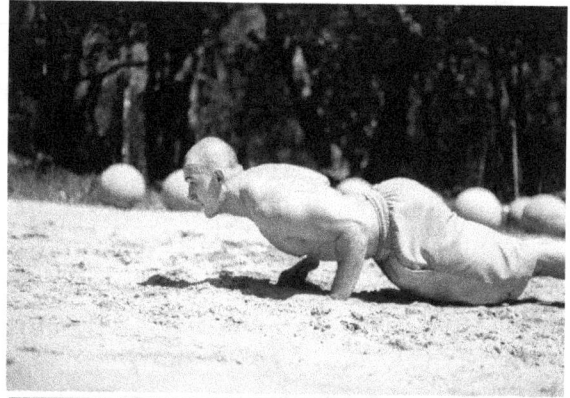

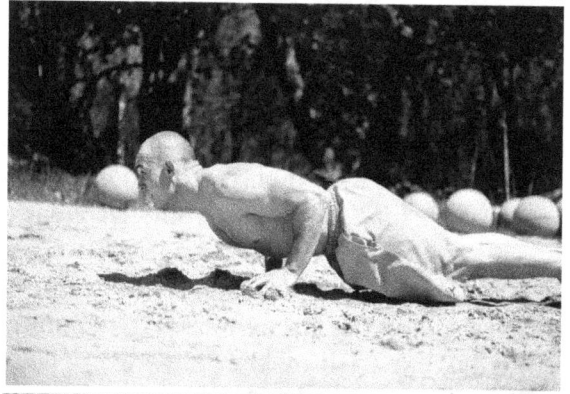

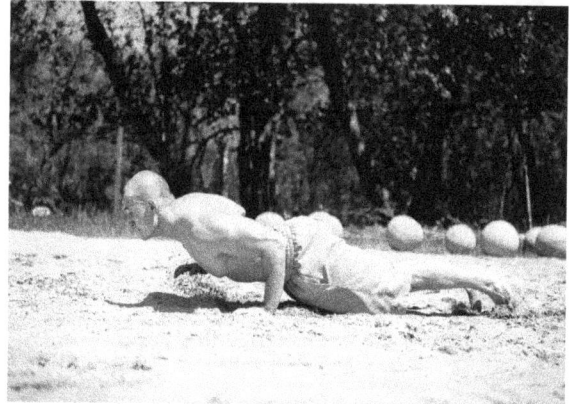

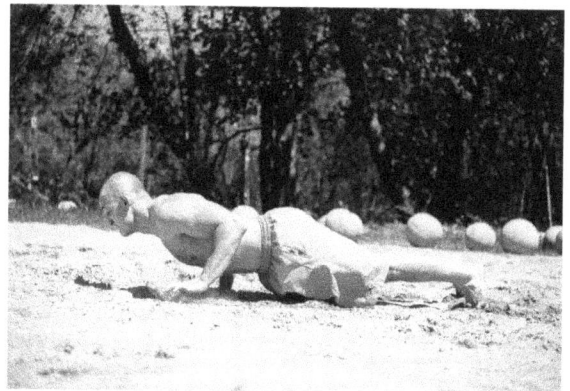

Depth Drop in the Sand

Classification: Power/Force Absorption/Upright Stability

Exercise Prerequisites: Four week familiarization and adaptation to sand training is recommended prior to engaging in high intensity jump training in the sand. You may want to avoid if you have Achilles tendon, knee, hip, low back, ankle, or neck issues.

Movement: These are not true depth drops with optimal plyometric effect due to the fact that the landing forces are dissipated through the sand, rather than the athlete's musculotendinous chain. For that reason we have chosen to name them accordingly (non-plyometric). To perform a non-true plyometric Depth Drop in the sand, stand on a box, bench, or other elevated platform (the height to be determined by training experience/ lower extremity strength or vertical jump height). Step forward and fall off the platform. Depending on your strength levels and training experience you may also try jumping upward and outward off the platform, kicking your knees high. If dropping off the platform you should aim to fall out roughly the distance equal to the height of the box. Land softly in the sand, minimizing knee bend and torso flexion. Trying not to allow the weight to shift completely to your heels upon impact. Stick the landing for 3-5 seconds. As these are done in the sand, athletes may not have to take the recommended minimum of 1-minute rest between each drop.

Keys to Movement:

1. Stand on an optimal box height according to your training experience, strength levels, and vertical jump height.
2. Drop off the platform and stick the landing softly on both feet with minimal flexion at the knees and hips.
3. Hold landing for 3-5 seconds.

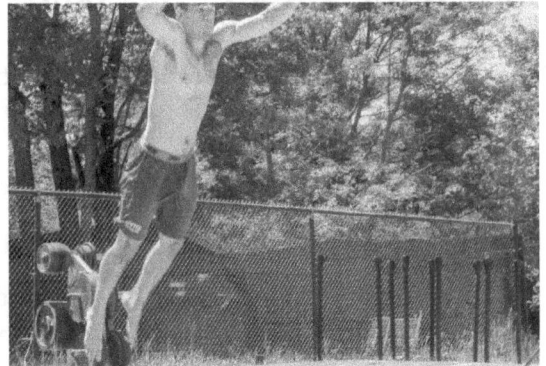

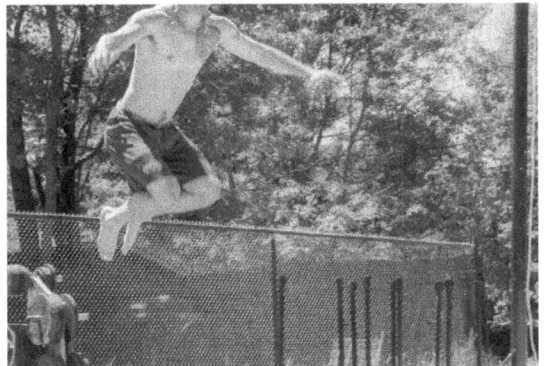

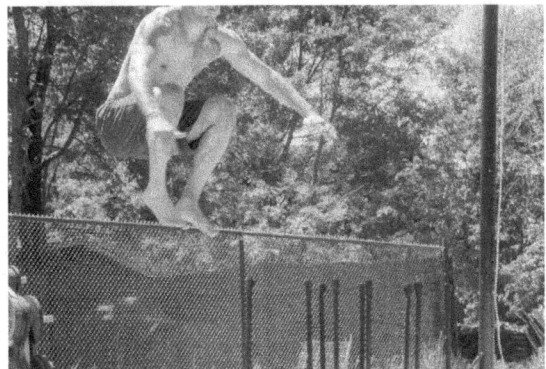

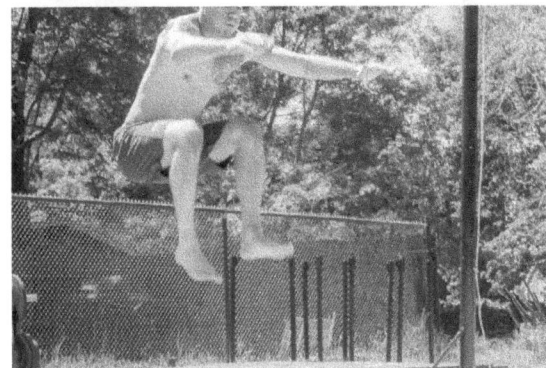

Depth Drop To Sprint in the Sand

Classification: Power and speed development

Exercise Prerequisites: Avoid if chronic neck, knee, shoulder or low back pain.

Movement: Perform a depth drop and immediately sprint a predetermined distance. Pausing for 1-3 seconds in the landing position is an option.

Keys to Movement:

1. Maintain torso stability while minimizing knee bend on the landing.
2. Pause or immediately sprint upon landing.

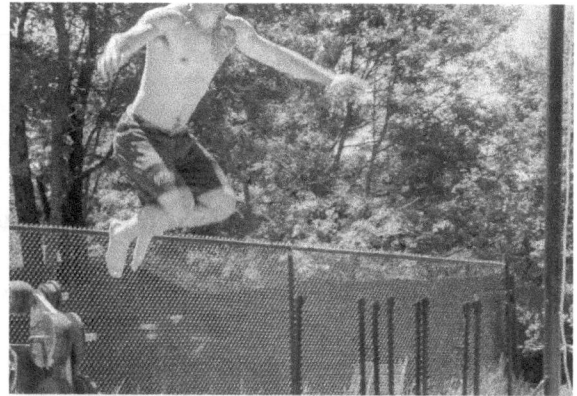

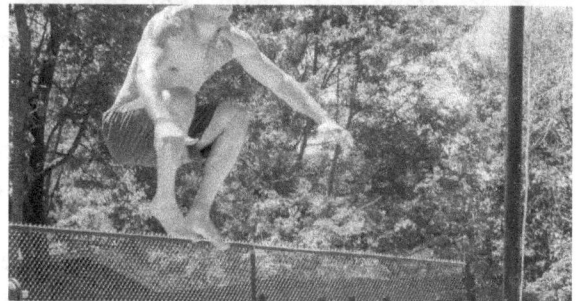

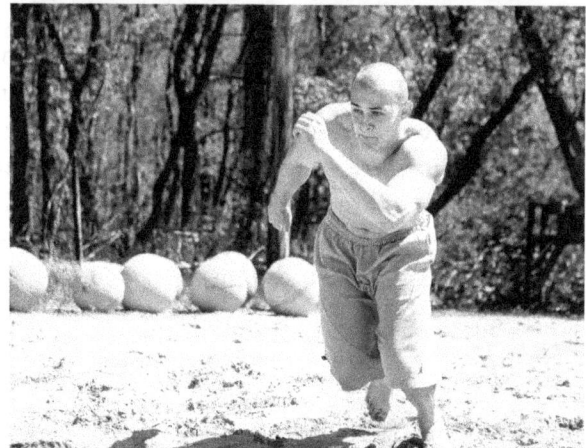

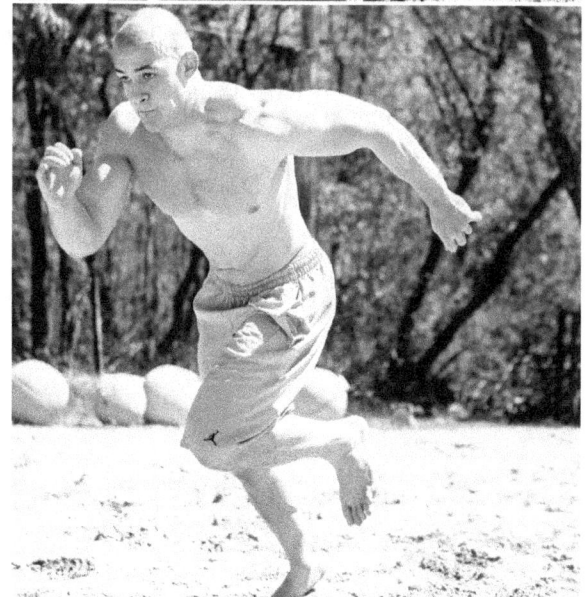

Depth Jump in the Sand

Exercise Prerequisites: Four week familiarization and adaptation to sand training is recommended prior to engaging in high intensity jump training in the sand. You may want to avoid if you have Achilles tendon, knee, hip, low back, ankle, or neck issues.

Movement: These are not true depth jumps with optimal plyometric effect due to the fact that the landing forces are dissipated through the sand, rather than the athlete's musculotendinous chain. For this reason we have chosen to name them accordingly (non-plyometric). To perform a non-true plyometric Depth Jump in the sand stand on a box (the height to be determined by training experience/lower extremity strength or actual vertical jump height) with hands behind you in the propulsive phase position of jumping. Step forward and fall off the box. You should fall out roughly the same distance as the height of the box. (If you are standing on a 24" box you should land roughly 24" away from the box). Think about jumping before you land. A good tip is to think of the ground as a hot stove as you will burn your feet if you are on the ground for too long. As soon as you land, minimize knee bend, hip flexion, torso flexion, and heel contact with the ground. Immediately jump up, swinging the arms upward while extending at the hips, knees, ankles, and torso

Keys to Movement:

1. Stand on an optimal box height according to your training experience, strength levels, and vertical jump height.
2. Drop off the platform and land with feet hip width and parallel.
3. Try to minimize knee bend, hip flexion, torso flexion, and ground contact time.
4. Immediately reverse direction, swing your arms upward, and jump as high as you can into the air.

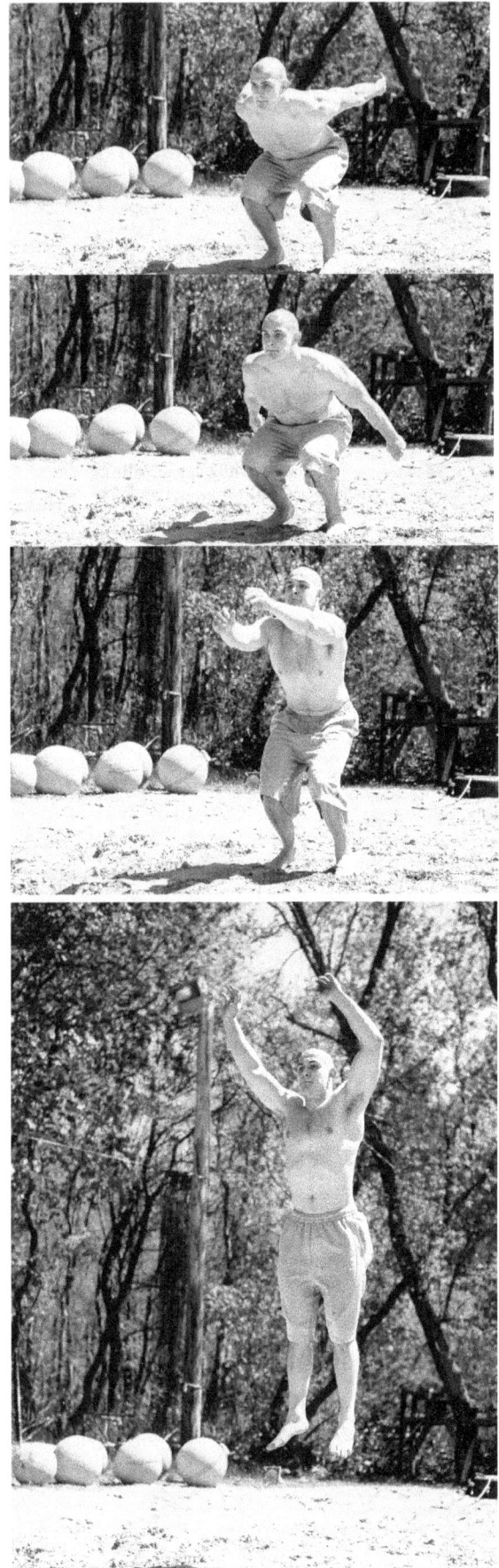

Depth Jump To Squat Throw in the Sand

Classification: Total Body Power

Exercise Prerequisites: Avoid if chronic neck, knee, shoulder or low back pain.

Movement: Holding a medicine ball in a chest pass position, drop into a depth jump. Upon landing, immediately reverse direction and explode into a chest pass medicine ball throw.

Keys to Movement:

1. Hold me ball in chest pass throw position.
2. Minimize ground contact time and explode into chest pass med ball throw.

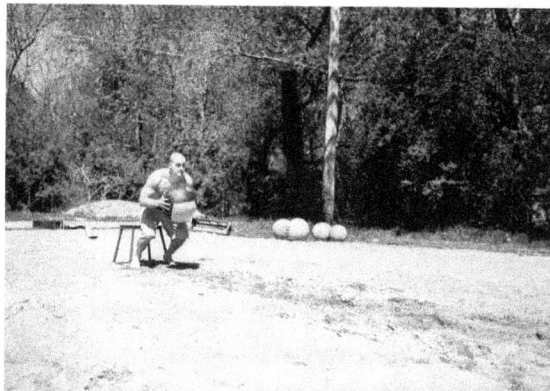

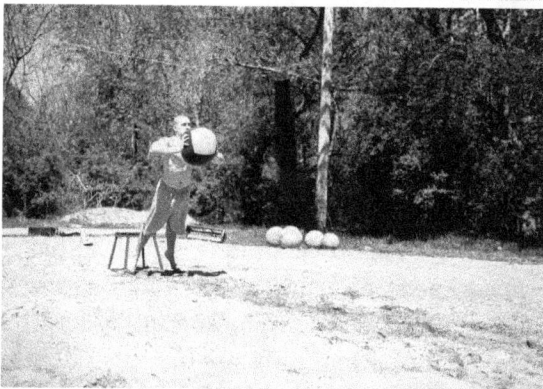

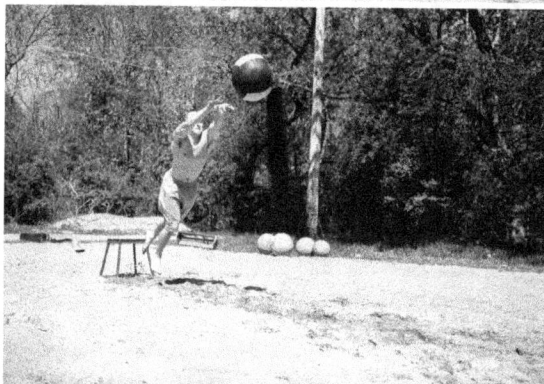

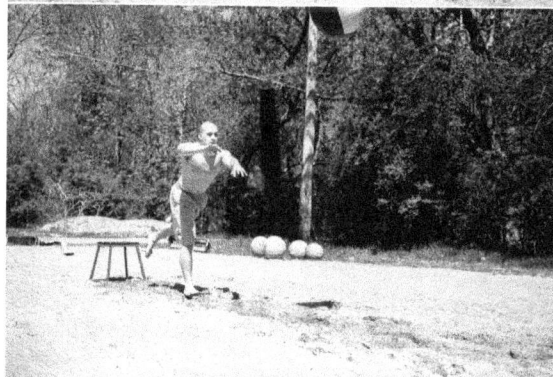

Farmer Carry Backward in the sand

Classification: Total Body Strength, Stability, and Conditioning

Exercise Prerequisites: Avoid if chronic neck, knee, shoulder or low back pain.

Movement: Similar to the farmer carry forward, but walking backwards. Once you have ensured there are no obstacles or large holes, face away from the sand trail. Begin by placing implements of your choice by your sides. These may include farmer carry hands, kettlebells, dumbbells, water buckets, etc. Holding neutral to lordotic back posture, with feet either slightly staggered or parallel to each other, and knees bent, reach place hands on implement handles, Lift using proper deadlift technique. Once stable begin walking backwards, focusing on keeping torso upright, arms by your sides, chest high, and shoulders tense. Creating intra-abdominal pressure may also help in keeping the torso rigid and upright. Walk for predetermined time or distance.

Keys to Movement:

1. Lift implements with proper deadlift technique.
2. Maintain intra-abdominal pressure to stabilize rigid posture.
3. Keep chest high and shoulders tense to maintain posture.
4. Walk for predetermined time or distance.

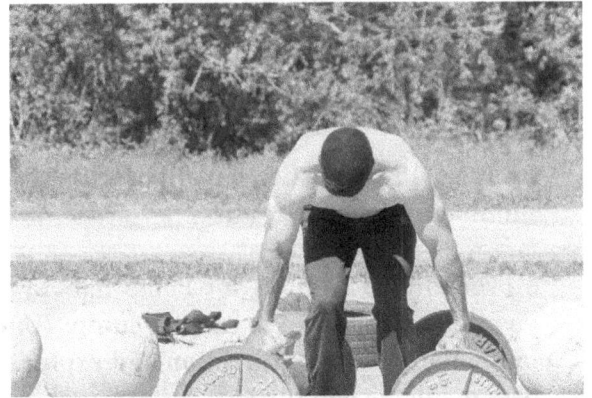

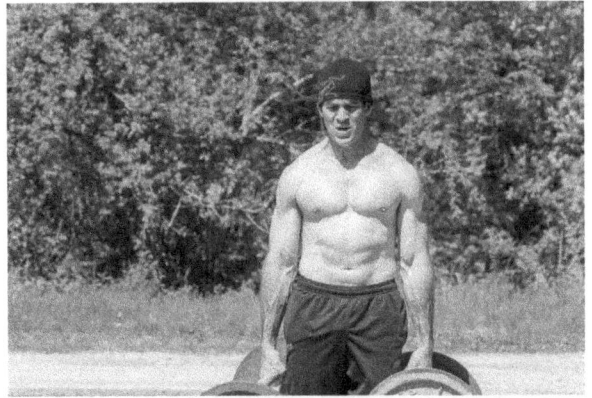

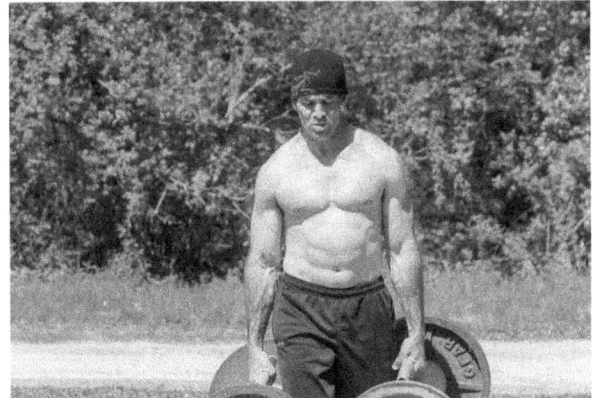

Farmer Carry Forward

Classification: Total Body Strength, Stability, and Conditioning

Exercise Prerequisites: Avoid if chronic neck, knee, shoulder or low back pain.

Movement: Begin by placing implements of your choice by your sides. These may include farmer carry hands, kettlebells, dumbbells, water buckets, etc. Holding neutral to lordotic back posture, with feet either slightly staggered or parallel to each other, and knees bent, reach place hands on implement handles, Lift using proper deadlift technique. Once stable begin walking, focusing on keeping torso upright, arms by your sides, chest high, and shoulders tense. Creating intra-abdominal pressure may also help in keeping the torso rigid and upright. Walk for predetermined time or distance.

Keys to Movement:

1. Lift implements with proper deadlift technique.
2. Maintain intra-abdominal pressure to stabilize rigid posture.
3. Keep chest high and shoulders tense to maintain posture.
4. Walk for predetermined time or distance.

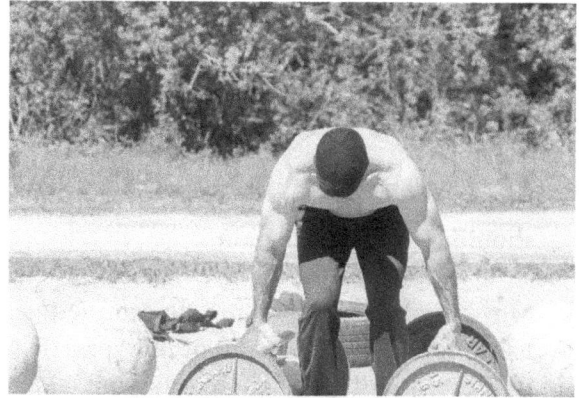

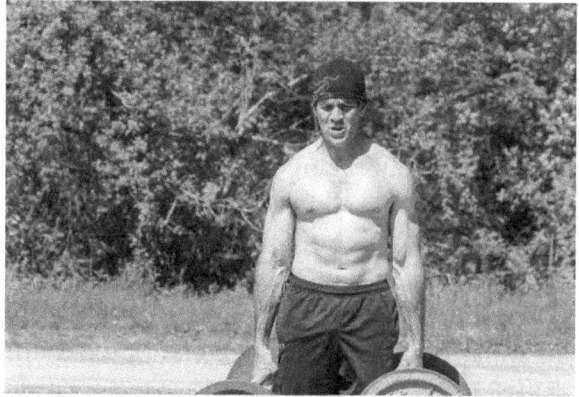

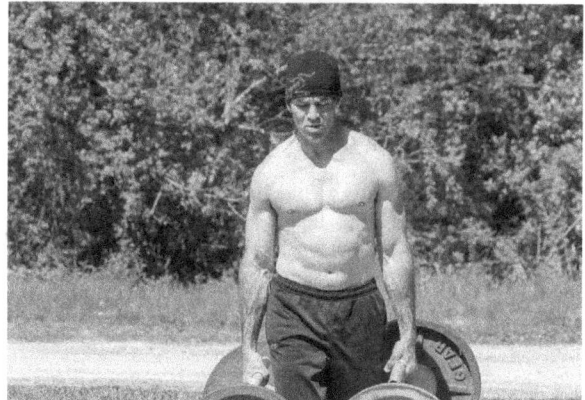

Farmer Carry Slalom

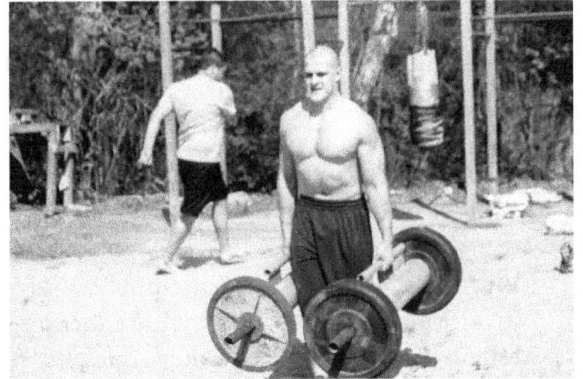

Classification: Total Body Strength, Stability, and Conditioning

Exercise Prerequisites: Avoid if chronic neck, knee, shoulder or low back pain.

Movement: Set up a pre-determined slalom course using cones or other types of markers. Begin by placing implements of your choice by your sides. These may include farmer carry hands, kettlebells, dumbbells, water buckets, etc. Holding neutral to lordotic back posture, with feet either slightly staggered or parallel to each other, and knees bent, reach place hands on implement handles, Lift using proper deadlift technique. Once stable begin walking around each marker, focusing on keeping torso upright, arms by your sides, chest high, and shoulders tense. Creating intra-abdominal pressure may also help in keeping the torso rigid and upright. Walk through slalom course for predetermined time or distance.

Keys to Movement:

1. Lift implements with proper deadlift technique.
2. Maintain intra-abdominal pressure to stabilize rigid posture.
3. Keep chest high and shoulders tense to maintain posture.
4. Walk for predetermined time or distance.

Forward Backward Jumps in the Sand

Classification: Total Body Power/Agility

Exercise Prerequisites: Avoid if chronic knee, shoulder, neck or low back pain.

Movement: Using a downward counter movement, jump over a desired obstacle. Upon landing, minimize ground contact time and proceed to jump backward over the object.

Keys to Movement:

1. Utilize countermovement to jump over low object.
2. Upon landing, minimize ground contact time and jump backward back over the object.

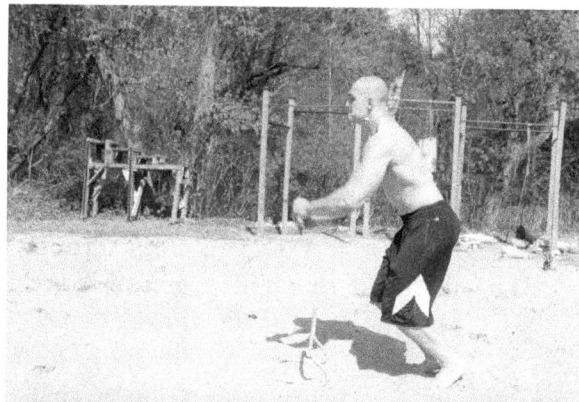

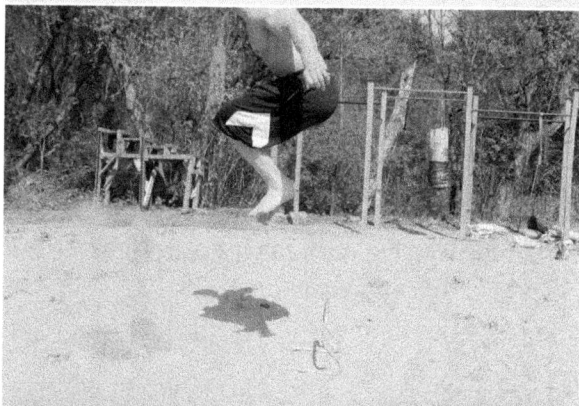

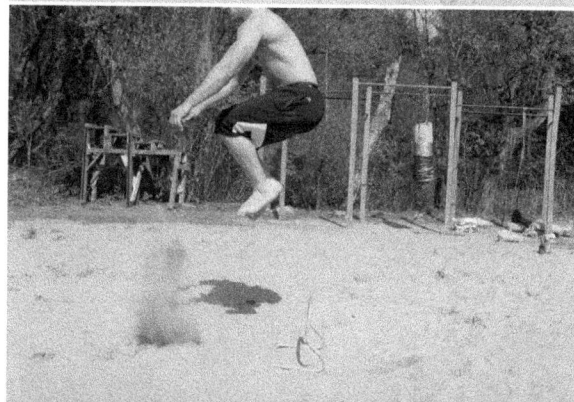

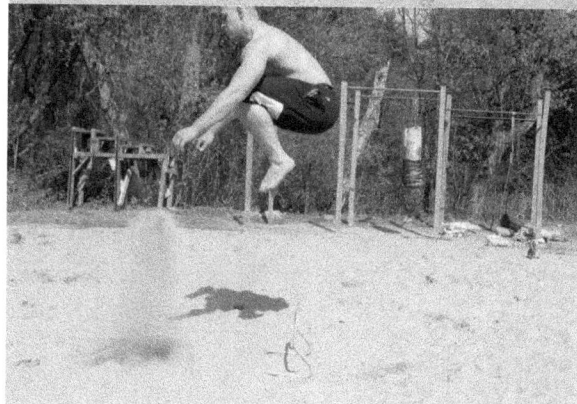

Forward Sled Dragging in the Sand

Classification: Lower Body Strength and Conditioning

Exercise Prerequisites: Four week familiarization and adaptation to sand training is recommended prior to engaging in high intensity jump training in the sand. You may want to avoid if you have Achilles tendon, knee, hip, low back, ankle, or neck issues.

Movement: Facing away from a sled, holding the straps by your sides with arms extended. Lean forward to roughly 45 degree angle relative to the floor. Feet should be feet hip width apart. Keeping the same torso position with arms straight by your sides, begin walking by driving the knee upward and landing in a modified lunge. From here focus on pulling with the hip extensors of the lead leg until the leg is straight. Drive the opposite knee high and repeat.

Keys to Movement:

1. Position feet hip width apart.
2. Lean over with torso roughly 45 degrees relative to the floor.
3. Keep arms extended by your sides.
4. Lunge step outward, driving the lead leg knee high.
5. Focus on driving forward using the lead leg hip extensor musculature.

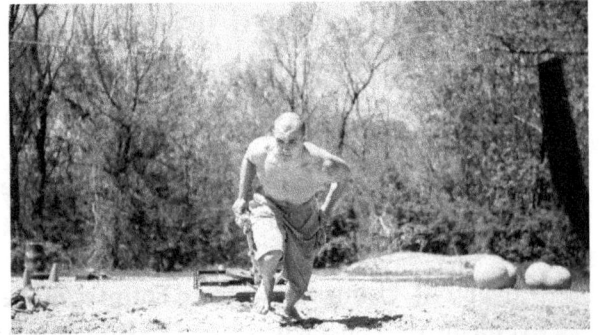

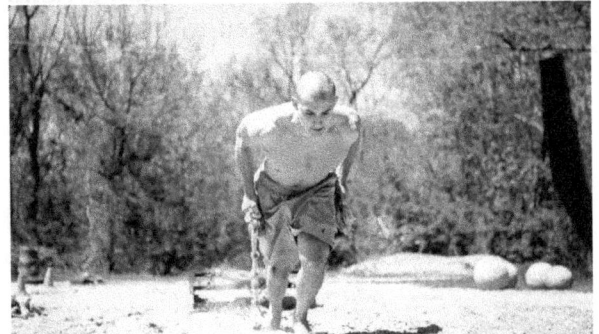

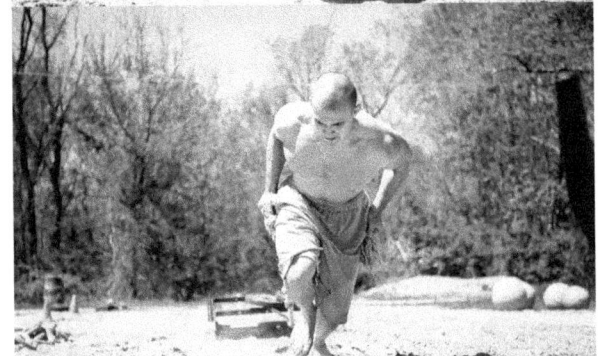

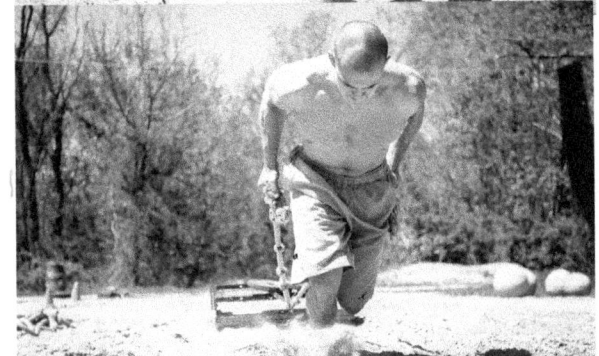

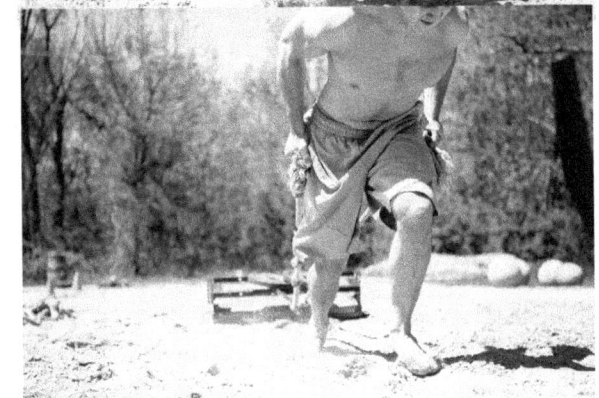

Hand Over Hand Atlas Stone Pull

Classification: Total Body Functional Strength and Conditioning

Exercise Prerequisites: Avoid if chronic neck, knee, shoulder or low back pain.

Antagonistic Exercises: Hand Over Hand Atlas Stone Push, Pressing Movements, Internal Rotator Exercises

Movement: Begin with feet wide and hand on the far side of the atlas stone. Pull the stone toward you with one arm at a time while extending back. Shuffle backward, keeping your feet wide as the ball begins to roll.

Keys to Movement:

1. Start with two hands on the far side of the atlas stone with knees bent and feet wide.
2. Pull the stone through toward you through your legs while extending your back.
3. Shuffle feet back to the sides of the stone and reset.
4. Aim for quality of movement first, then try to increase speed or weight of the stone.

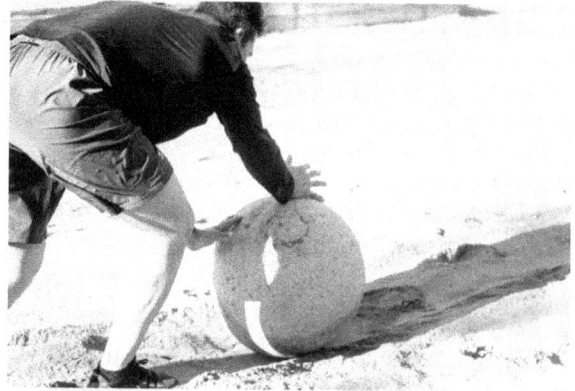

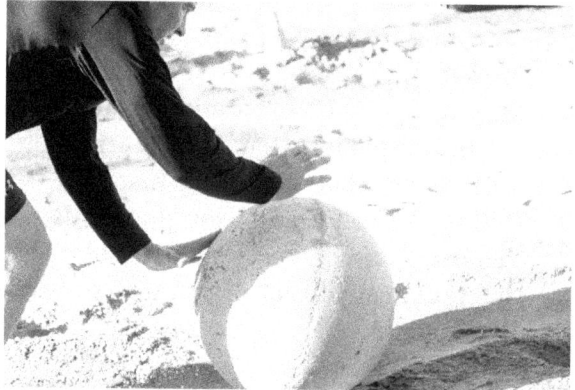

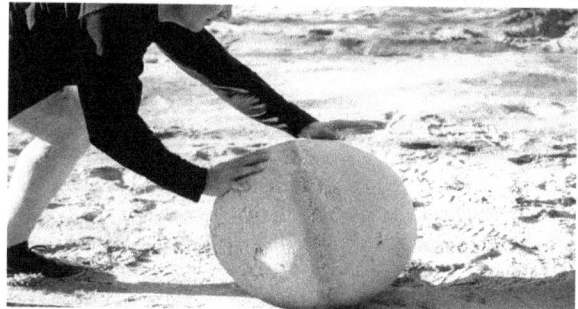

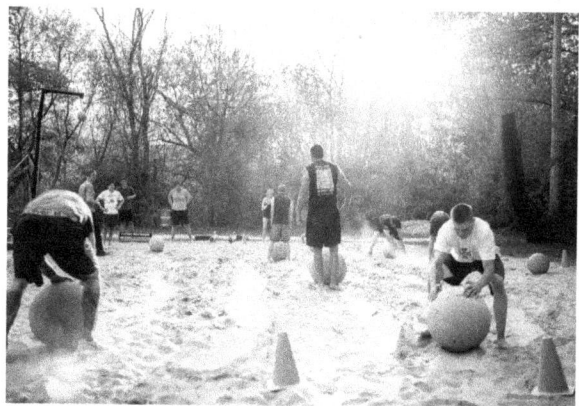

Hand Over Hand Atlas Stone Push

Classification: Total Body Functional Strength and Conditioning

Exercise Prerequisites: Avoid if chronic neck, knee, shoulder or low back pain.

Antagonistic Exercises: Hand Over Hand Atlas Stone Pull, Hand Over Hand Rope Pull, Row Movements, External Rotator Exercises, Mid Trapezius Exercises

Movement: Position your hands on an atlas stone with knees bent and torso parallel (or close to parallel) to the ground. Begin by extending one arm, re-positioning the other hand, then extending that arm to get the stone rolling. As you are driving the hands, walk or shuffle the feet, keeping your torso parallel to the floor. Drive the stone around each of the cones for time, distance, or stone weight.

Keys to Movement:

1.   Start with two hands on atlas stone with knees bent and torso parallel to the ground.
2.   Extend one arm pushing the stone forward.
3.   Switch hands and extend other arm continuing the push.
4.   Maintain torso as parallel as possible to the ground.
5.   Quickly shuffle feet to keep the ball moving forward.
6.   Aim for quality of movement first, then try to increase speed or weight of the stone.

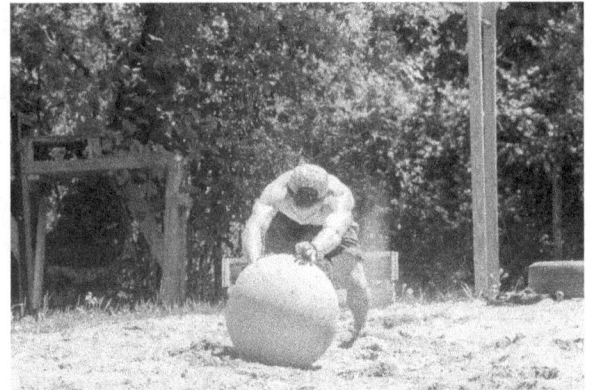

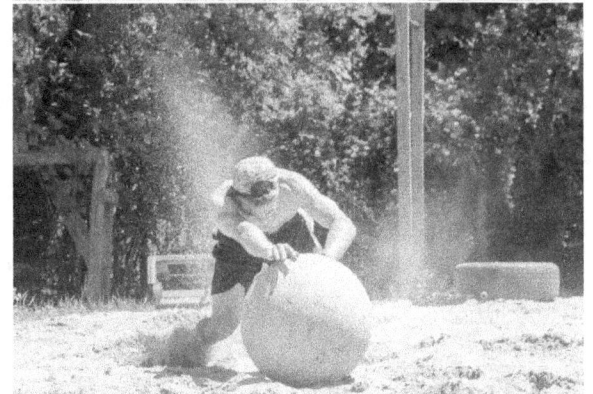

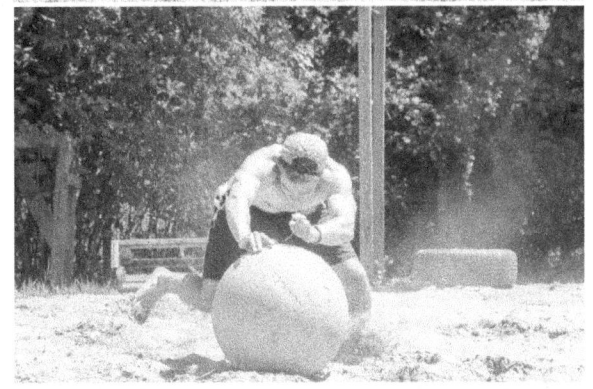

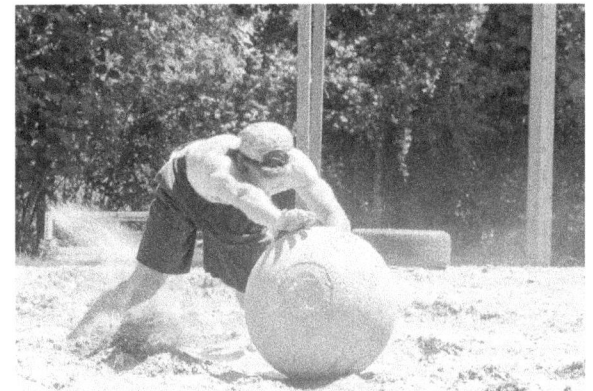

Hand Over Hand Atlas Stone Slalom Push

Classification: Total Body Functional Strength and Conditioning

Exercise Prerequisites: Avoid if chronic neck, knee, shoulder or low back pain.

Antagonistic Exercises: Hand Over Hand Atlas Stone Pull, Hand Over Hand Rope Pull, Row Movements, External Rotator Exercises, Mid Trapezius Exercises

Movement: Set up a slalom course using cones. Distance and angle between cones is your preference. Position your hands on an atlas stone with knees bent and torso parallel (or close to parallel) to the ground. Begin by extending one arm, re-positioning the other hand, then extending that arm to get the stone rolling. As you are driving the hands, walk or shuffle the feet, keeping your torso parallel to the floor. Drive the stone around each of the cones for time, distance, or stone weight.

Keys to Movement:

1. Start with two hands on atlas stone with knees bent and torso parallel to the ground.
2. Extend one arm pushing the stone forward.
3. Switch hands and extend other arm continuing the push.
4. Maintain torso as parallel as possible to the ground.
5. Quickly shuffle feet to keep the ball moving forward.
6. Aim for quality of movement first, then try to increase speed or weight of the stone.

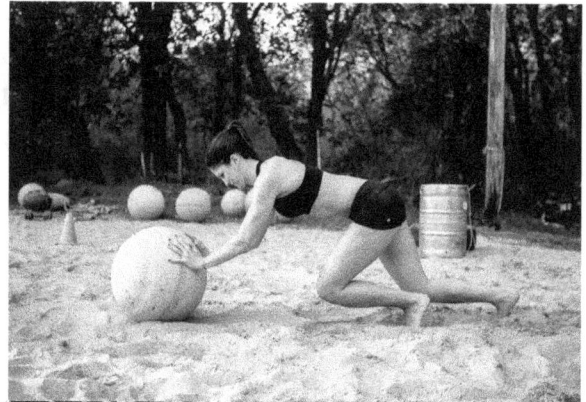

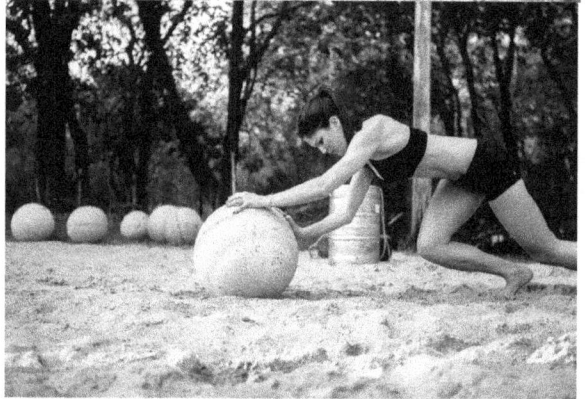

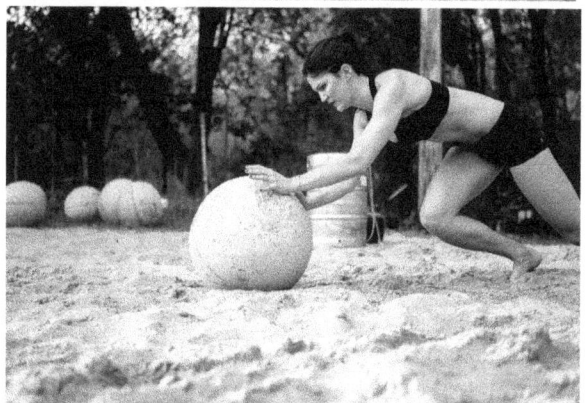

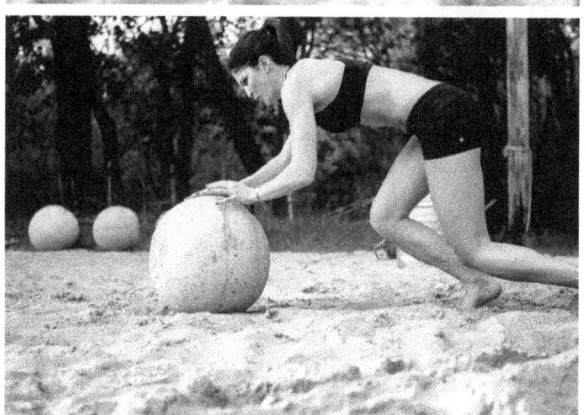

Hand Over Hand Rope Pull

Classification: Total Body Functional Strength and Conditioning

Exercise Prerequisites: Avoid if chronic neck, knee, shoulder or low back pain.

Movement: Attach a rope to a sled, Heavy bag, or other implement and extend the rope. Sit or stand at the opposite end of the rope. With one hand over the other, begin pulling the rope toward you, alternating hands. Variations may include short pulls, longer pulls, two handed pulls, spinal and hip extension pulls, and elbows high pulls.

Keys to Movement:

1. Safety needs to be paramount. If you have back, shoulder, or elbow issues you may want to forego this exercise.
2. If healthy, feel free to experiment with the different variations of this exercise.

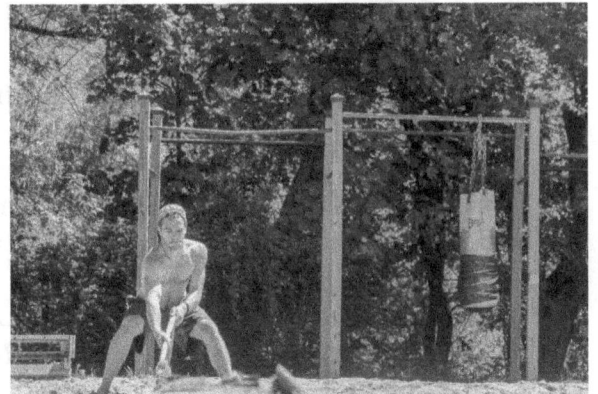

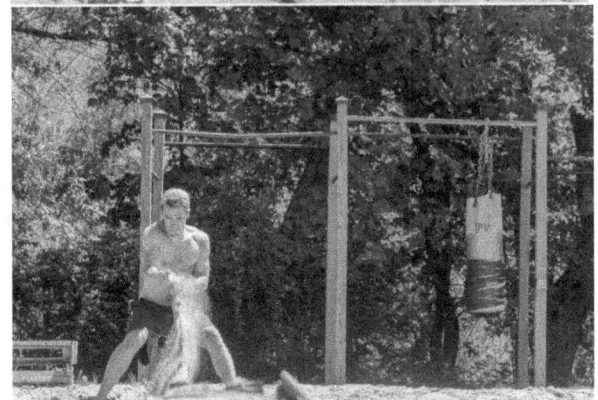

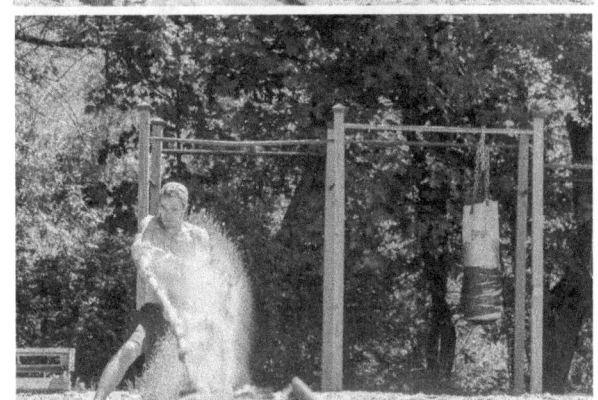

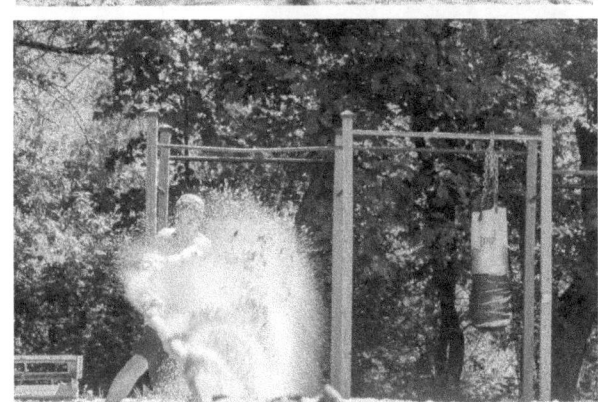

Heavy Bag Carry

Classification: Total Body Functional Strength and Conditioning

Exercise Prerequisites: Avoid if chronic neck, knee, shoulder or low back pain.

Movement: This is a great exercise for strengthening the muscles of the core, hips, low and mid back, grip, and elbow flexors. Begin by placing the heavy bag upright in front of you. Try holding a neutral to lordotic back posture to lift the bag, (though you may need to allow for a kyphotic lifting posture), with feet wide and parallel to each other. Keeping your knees slightly bent, "bear hug" the bag and lock your hands together or grab your wrist on the opposite side. Lift the back with optimal posture and walk for predetermined time or distance. Try to maintain rigid upright torso posture. Other carry options include over one shoulder, on the hip, or horizontal in front.

Keys to Movement:

1. Lift heavy bag with your optimal lifting technique for this object.
2. "Bear hug" the bag and lock the hands together or grab a wrist on the opposite side of the bag.
3. Try to maintain rigid upright torso posture.
4. Walk for predetermined time or distance.

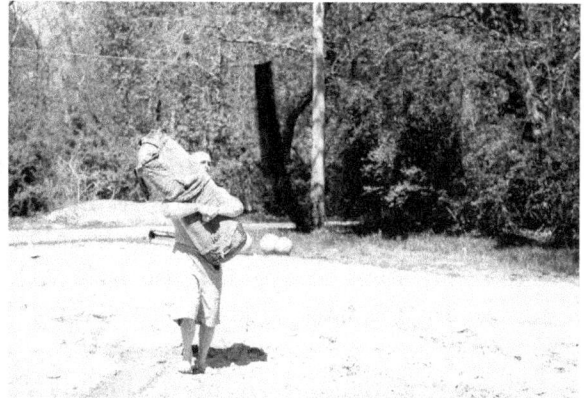

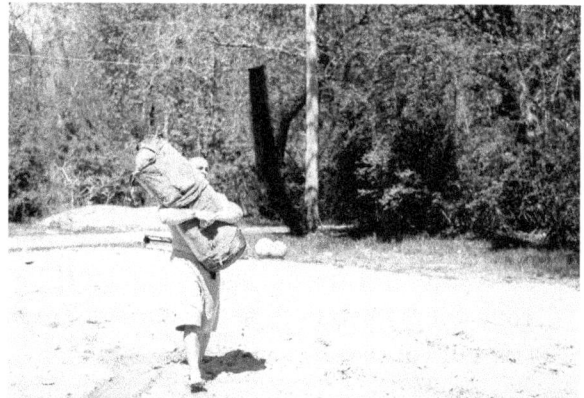

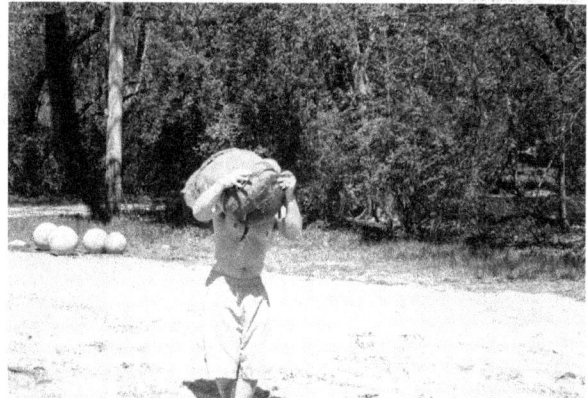

High Hurdle Hops in the Sand

Classification: Total Body Power

Exercise Prerequisites: Four week familiarization and adaptation to sand training is recommended prior to engaging in high intensity jump training in the sand. You may want to avoid if you have Achilles tendon, knee, hip, low back, ankle, or neck issue

Movement: Set up at the most 5 high (greater than 12") hurdles roughly 2-4 feet apart. Standing erect, with feet hip width apart and toes pointing forward or slightly out, jump as high as you can over the hurdle pulling your knees to your chest to clear your feet over the hurdle. Once you land, try to minimize ground contact time and jump as high as you can over the next hurdle, once again pulling your knees toward your chest. Make sure your feet do not kick your butt, instead pulling your knees to your chest so your feet are slightly out in front of your body.

Keys to Movement:
1.   Keeping torso erect, jump as high as you can pulling your knees toward your chest to clear your feet over the hurdle.
2.   Utilize a countermovement arm swing with each jump.
3.   Land properly, minimize ground contact time, and jump again over the next hurdle.
4.   Make sure your feet do not kick your butt

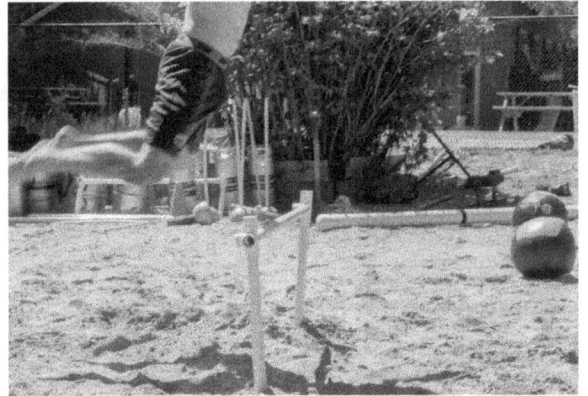

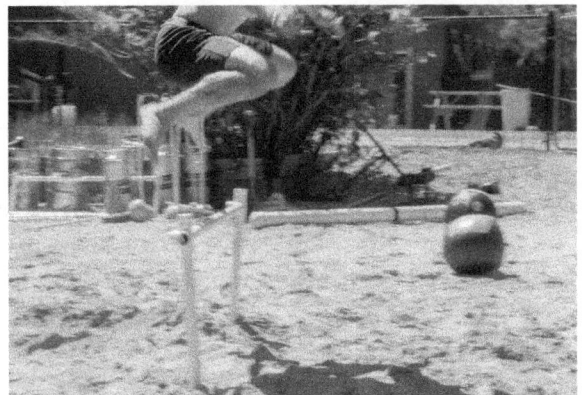

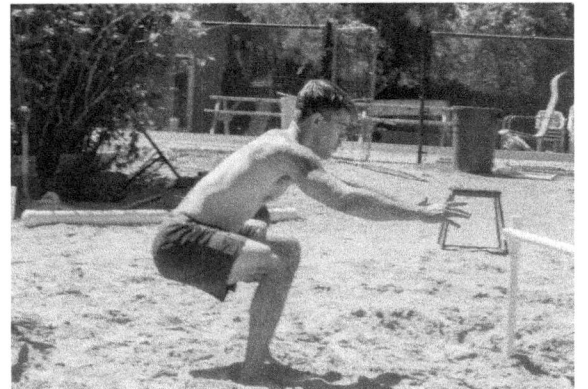

Ickey Shuffle Agility Ladder Drill in the Sand

Classification: Warm Up/Quickness

Exercise Prerequisites: Avoid if chronic neck, knee, shoulder or low back pain.

Movement: Stand on one side at the beginning of the agility ladder. Moving at an angle, step the foot closest into the first rung, then step the other foot into the rung, Then step the lead leg out of the ladder, followed by the trail leg. Then reverse direction into the next rung. Maintain upright stability while minimizing heel and ground contact times.

Keys to Movement:

1. Maintain upright stability throughout movement.
2. Minimize heel contact and ground contact times.

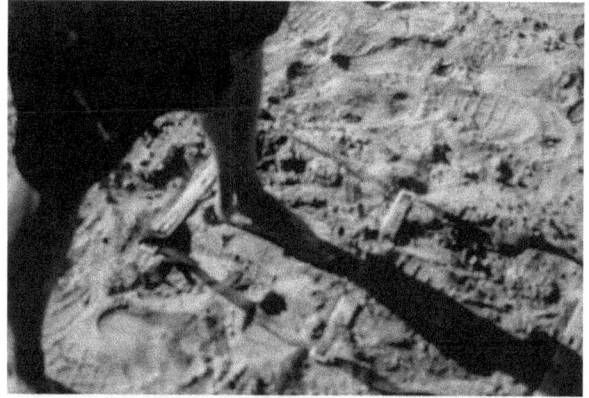

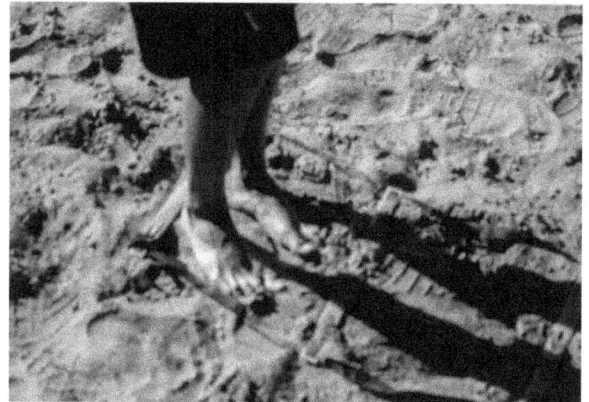

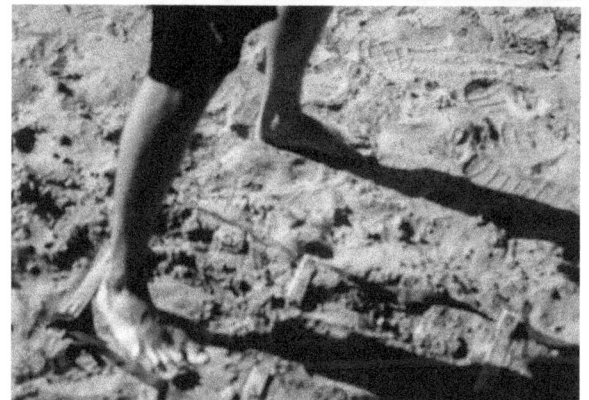

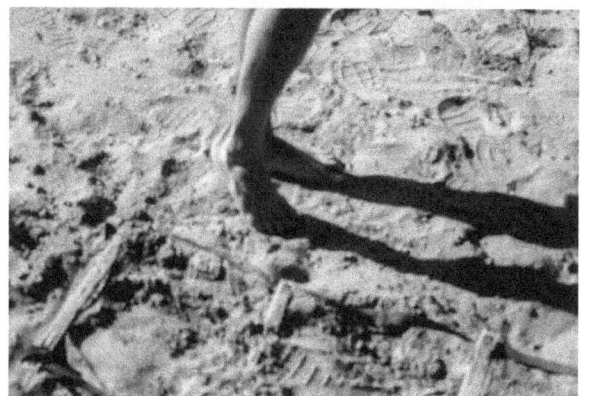

Inchworm in the sand

Exercise Prerequisites: Use caution if you have shoulder, low back, neck, elbow, wrist, or knee problems.

Movement: Start standing with legs straight and hand on ground in front of feet. Begin walking hand out as far as you are comfortable. Advanced athletes may walk out until nose or chest can touch the ground. Once you have walked out as far as comfortable, with straight legs, begin taking samll steps walking feet back toward hands. Continue for pre-determined distance or time.

Keys to Movement:

1. Start with legs straight and hand on ground in front of feet.
2. Walk hands out as far as comfortable.
3. Walk feet to hands and continue for pre-determined distance or time.

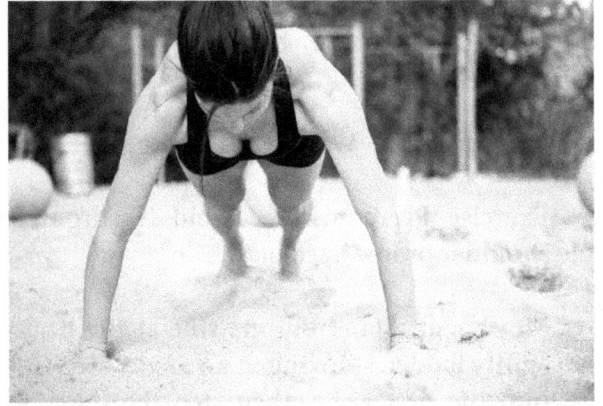

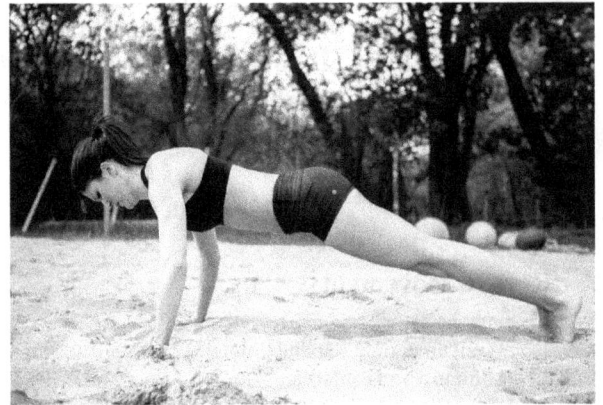

Illinois Agility Drill in the Sand

Classification: Agility

Exercise Prerequisites: Avoid if chronic neck, knee, shoulder or low back pain.

Movement: Place 4 cones in a rectangle, with the cones that make up the top and bottom of the rectangle 5 yards apart, and the cones that make the side of the rectangle 10 yards apart. Place 4 more cones down the length in the center of the rectangle. Make sure these are equidistant. The test starts with the athlete either lying down on the stomach or in a track or 40-start position at the first cone. The athlete sprint the 10 yard distance, then weaves down and back through the cones and sprint 10 more yards to the finish.

Keys to Movement:

1. Complete the drill as fast as you can.

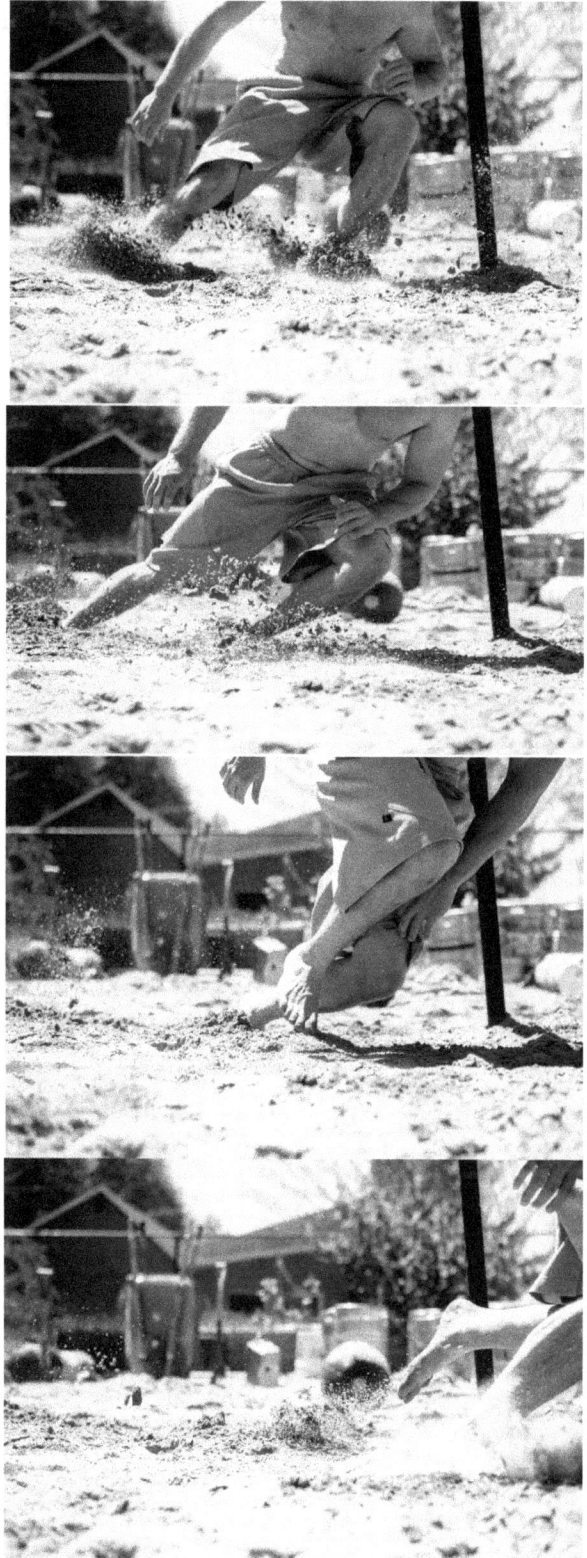

In And Out Agility Ladder Drill in the Sand

Classification: Warm-up/Quickness

Exercise Prerequisites: Avoid if chronic neck, knee, shoulder or low back pain.

Movement: Stand on the side of the agility ladder facing the ladder. Step your lead foot into the first rung, followed by the trail foot. Then lead leg out, trail leg out, and move onto the next rung. Continue down the ladder.

Keys to Movement:

1. Minimize heel and ground contact times.
2. Maintain stable upright posture throughout drill.

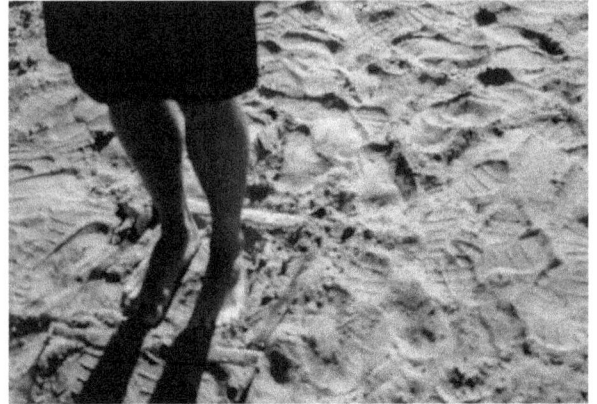

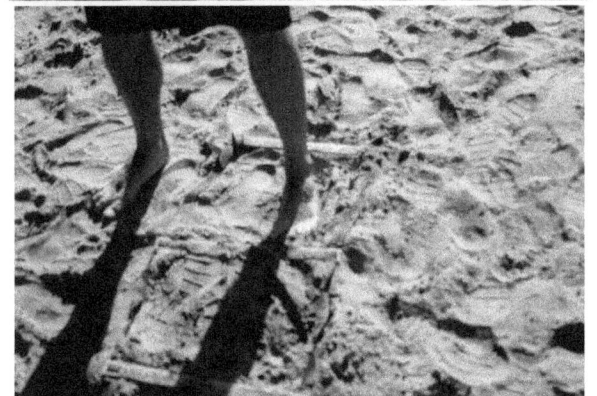

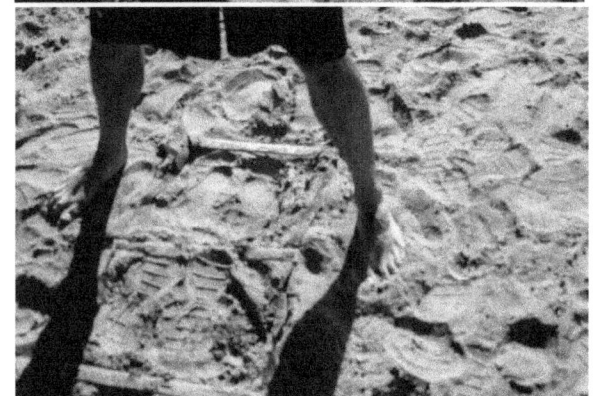

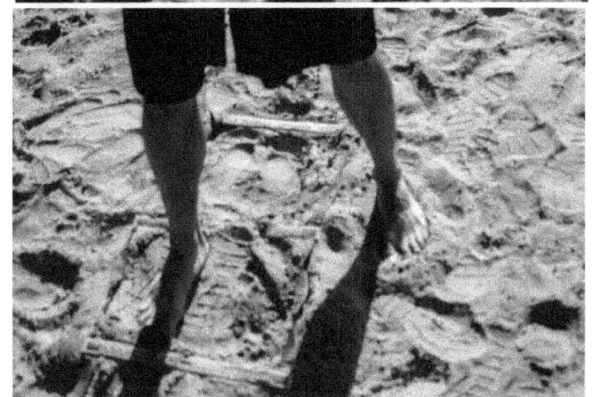

JumpBall Counter Step Jump in the Sand

Classification: Total Body Power Overhead Goal Training

Exercise Prerequisites: Four week familiarization and adaptation to sand training is recommended prior to engaging in high intensity jump training in the sand. You may want to avoid if you have Achilles tendon, knee, hip, low back, ankle, or neck issues.

Movement: Standing roughly 3-6 feet from the ball, take 1 to 2 powerful counter steps and perform a two legged vertical jump. Jump as high as possible to grab the ball or hit a vertical jump testing device. Land with optimal landing mechanics.

Movement Mechanics:

1. Start 3-6 feet from the Jumpball.
2. Take 1-2 powerful counter steps.
3. Vertical jump off of two feet grabbing the ball at a pre-determined height.
4. Land with optimal landing mechanics.

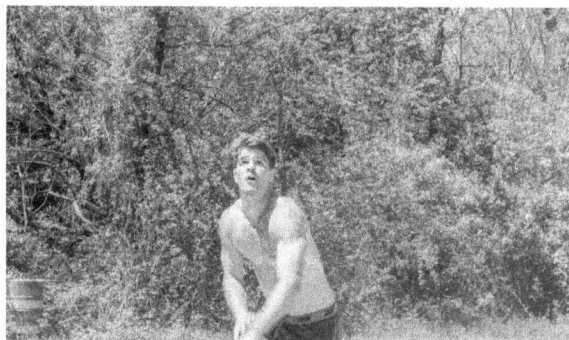

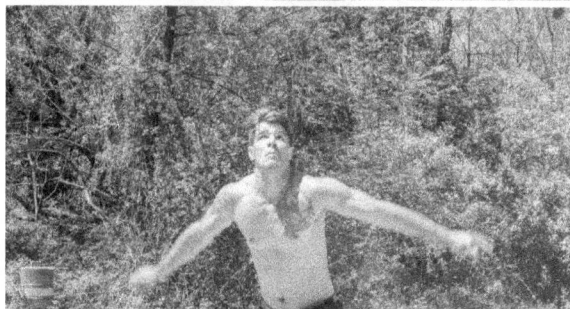

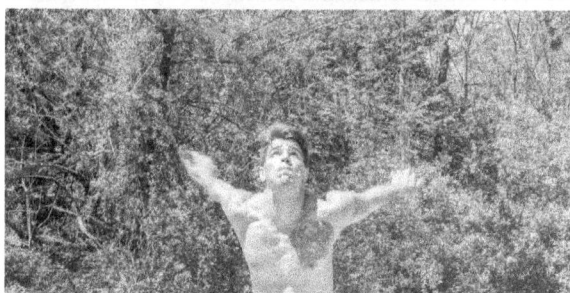

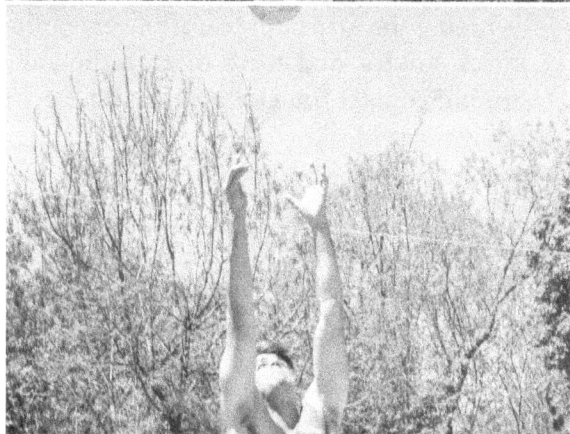

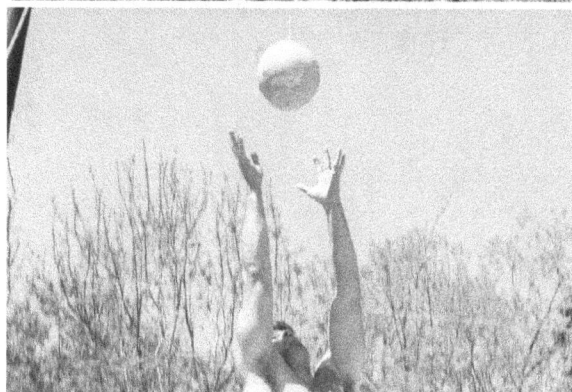

JumpBall Depth Jump in the Sand

Classification: Total Body Power Overhead Goal Training

Exercise Prerequisites: Four week familiarization and adaptation to sand training is recommended prior to engaging in high intensity jump training in the sand. You may want to avoid if you have Achilles tendon, knee, hip, low back, ankle, or neck issues.

Movement: Set up the Jumpball (can also use a vertec vertical jump tester) at a pre-determined height at a distance roughly equal to or slightly greater than the height of the box. Stand on a box (the height to be determined by training experience/lower extremity strength/ or actual vertical jump height) with your hands behind you in the propulsive phase position of jumping. Step forward and fall off box. You should fall out the distance equal to the height of the box. (If you are standing on a 24" box you should land 24" away from the box). Think about jumping before you land. (The ground is a hot stove so you will burn your feet if you are on the ground for too long.) As soon as you land, minimize knee bend, hip flexion, and do not let the heels touch the ground. Immediately jump up, swinging the arms upward while extending at the hips, knees, ankles, and torso to grab the ball. Try to keep ground contact time to less than one second, with .3-.5 being more ideal.

Keys to Movement:

1. Set up the Jumpball at a pre-determined. The distance between the box and the jumpball should be slightly greater than the height of the box you are dropping off.
2. Fall off the box, perform quick downward counter swing.
3. Immediately change direction and jump as high as you can trying to grab the ball or hit the height marker on the vertec.
4. Land with optimal landing mechanics.

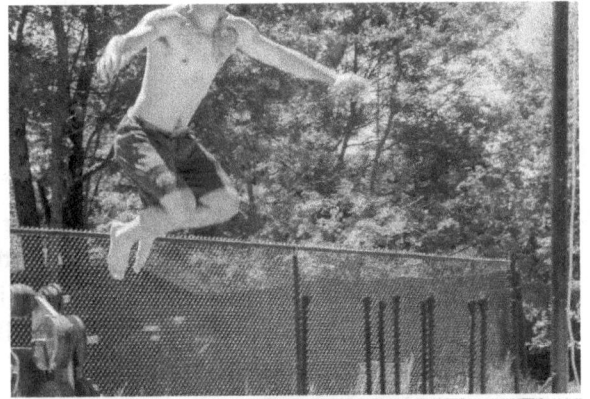

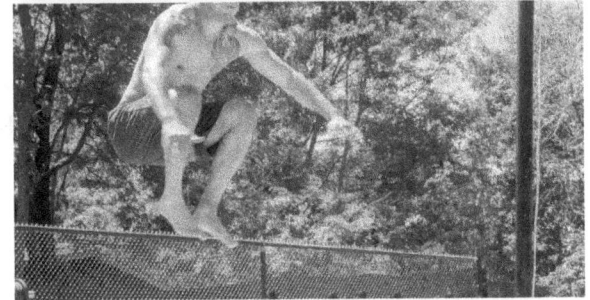

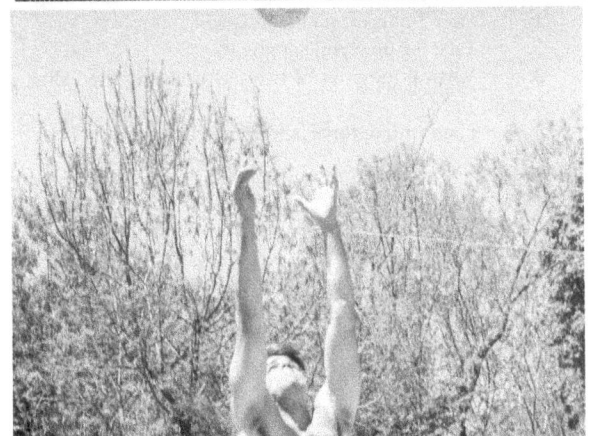

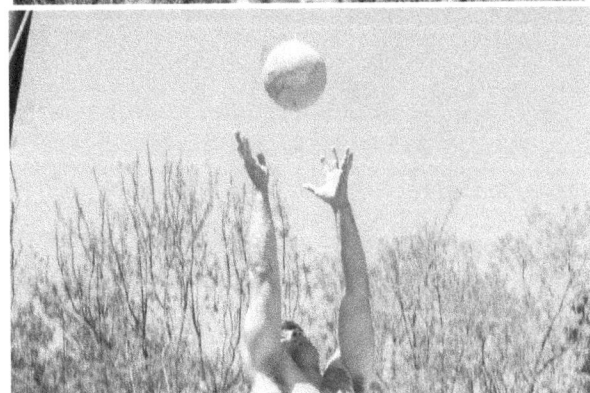

JumpBall Vertical Jumps in the Sand

Classification: Total Body Power Overhead Goal Training

Exercise Prerequisites: Four week familiarization and adaptation to sand training is recommended prior to engaging in high intensity jump training in the sand. You may want to avoid if you have Achilles tendon, knee, hip, low back, ankle, or neck issues.

Movement: Stand directly below the ball or 1-2 feet away with feet roughly hip width apart and toes pointing straight ahead. Perform vertical jump countermovement and jump as high as you can to grab the ball with both hands and pull it down with you. Once you have landed, release the ball, rest 5-10 seconds and repeat.

Keys to Movement:

1. Start directly below or 1-2 feet from the Jumpball.
2. Perform vertical jump countermovement.
3. Vertical jump off of two feet grabbing the ball at a pre-determined height.
4. Land with optimal landing mechanics.

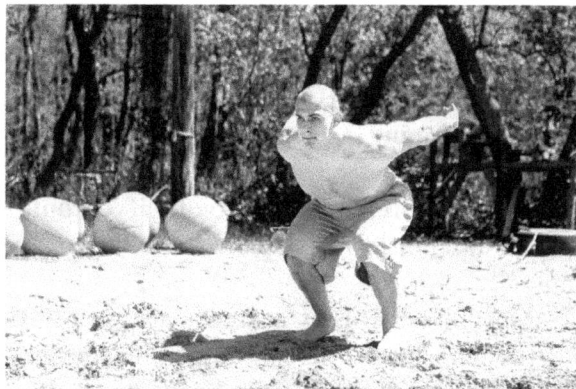

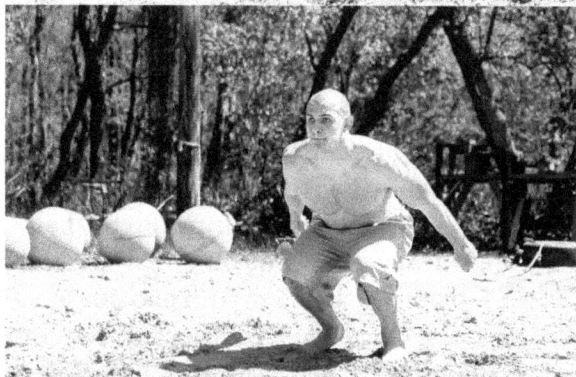

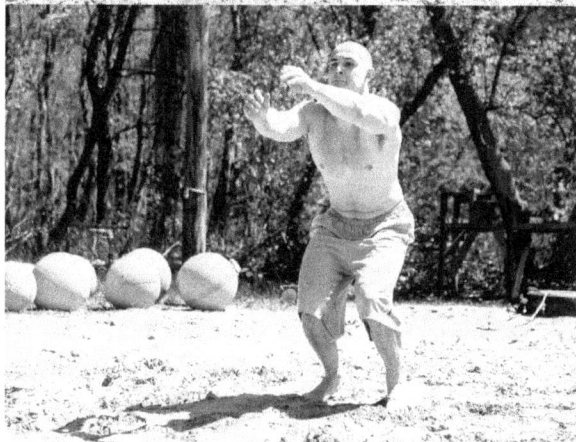

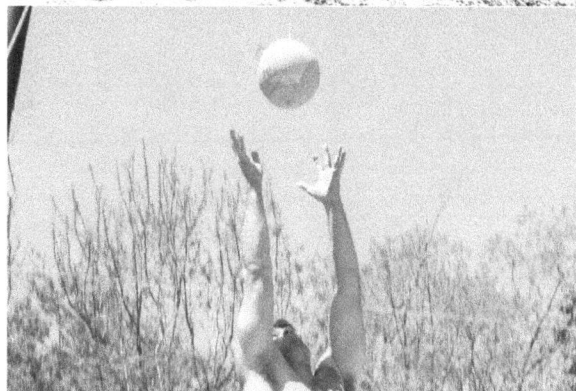

Keg Carry

Classification: Total Body Functional Strength and Conditioning

Exercise Prerequisites: Avoid if chronic neck, knee, shoulder or low back pain.

Movement: This is a great exercise for strengthening the muscles of the core, hips, low and mid back, grip, and elbow flexors. Begin by placing a keg on its side in front of you. Try to maintain a neutral to lordotic back posture to lift the keg, (though you may need to allow for a kyphotic lifting posture), with feet either wide or close depending on comfort level and body type. Keeping your knees slightly bent, lift the keg. Some athletes prefer to carry the keg above the hips/top of the thigh, holding both sides evenly, while other may prefer to hold above the hips/top of the thigh with one side much higher than the other. Once you have selected your optimal method of holding the keg, walk for predetermined time or distance. Try to maintain rigid upright torso posture.

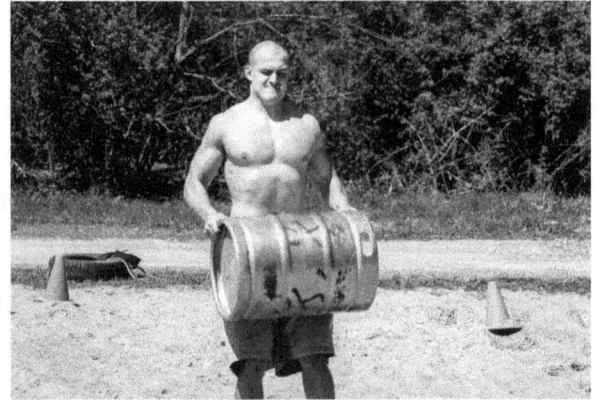

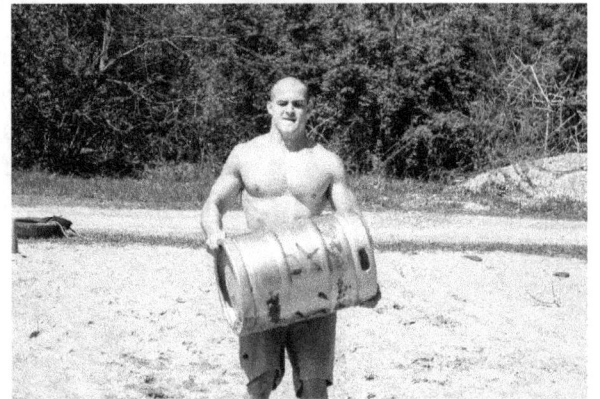

Keys to Movement:

1. Lift heavy keg with your optimal lifting technique for this object.
2. Try to carry keg at the top of the thigh or above the hips using your optimal carrying method.
3. Try to maintain rigid upright torso posture.
4. Walk for predetermined time or distance.

Lateral Skater Hops Over Low Hurdle

Classification: Unilateral Lower Body Power and Stability

Exercise Prerequisites: Four week familiarization and adaptation to sand training is recommended prior to engaging in high intensity jump training in the sand. You may want to avoid if you have Achilles tendon, knee, hip, low back, ankle, or neck issues.

Movement: Stand sideways roughly 1-2 feet from a low hurdle. Start on one leg with roughly 20-40 degree bend at knee and neutral to lordotic posture. Kick opposite leg behind you, flex the hip, and lean your torso out past your knee. Swing your arms downward and behind. At the point of optimal tension in the glutes and hamstrings, swing your arms upward jumping upward and sideways over the hurdle. Land with optimal landing mechanics on the opposite leg, keeping torso posture rigid. Perform same movement mechanics for other leg.

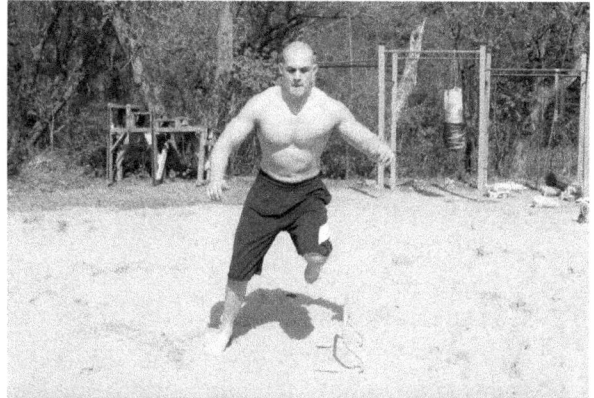

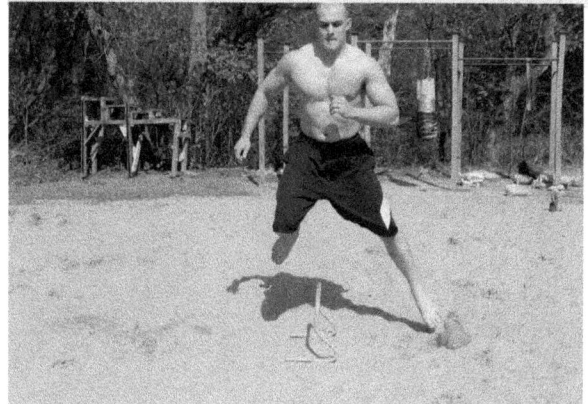

Keys to Movement:

1. Stand beside a low hurdle on one leg, keeping torso posture neutral/lordotic, and perform countermovement swing downward.
2. At point of optimal tension in glutes and hamstrings, swing arms upward and jump laterally over the hurdle onto the opposite leg.
3. Land with optimal landing mechanics and perform again with other leg.

Lateral High Knee Agility Ladder Drill in the Sand

Classification: Lateral Movement/Agility/Quickness

Exercise Prerequisites: Avoid if chronic neck, knee, shoulder or low back pain.

Movement: Start at one end of the ladder facing sideways. Perform high knees laterally, stepping each foot into each ladder rung. Maintain upright stable posture while minimizing ground contact time and heel contact.

Keys to Movement:

1. Maintain stable upright posture, keeping hips and shoulders squared.
2. Minimize ground contact time and heel contact.

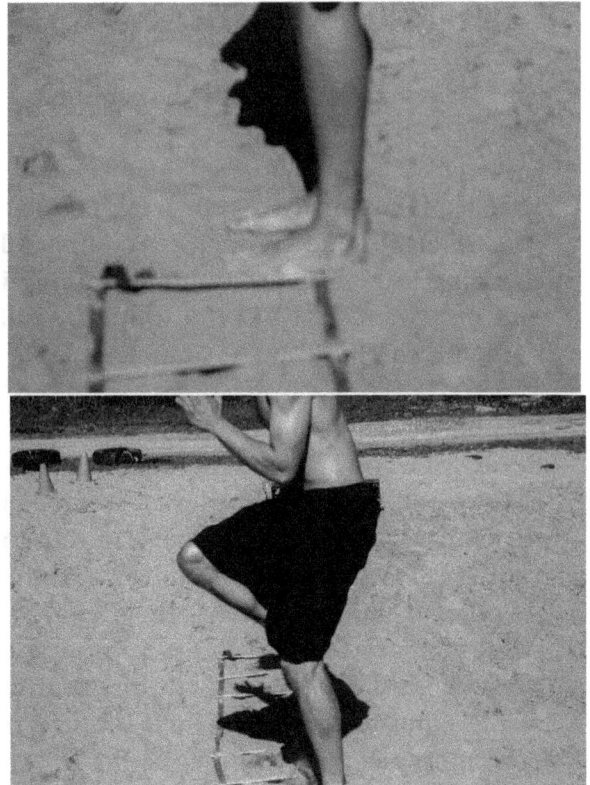

Lateral Plate Throw

Classification: Unilateral and Rotational Power

Exercise Prerequisites: Four week familiarization and adaptation to sand training is recommended prior to engaging in high intensity jump training in the sand. You may want to avoid if you have Achilles tendon, knee, hip, low back, ankle, or neck issues.

Movement: Hold a weight plat flat with palms facing each other and thumbs up. Position feet roughly shoulder width apart. Conter swing the plate roughly hip height in a rotational pattern toward your side and slighlty behind you. Powerfully swing and rotate your hips and torso throwing the plate as far as you can. Alternate sides for best results.

Keys to Movement:

1. Hold plate flat with palms facing each other and palms up.
2. Feet are roughly shoulder width apart.
3. Counter swing roughly hip height slightly behind you.

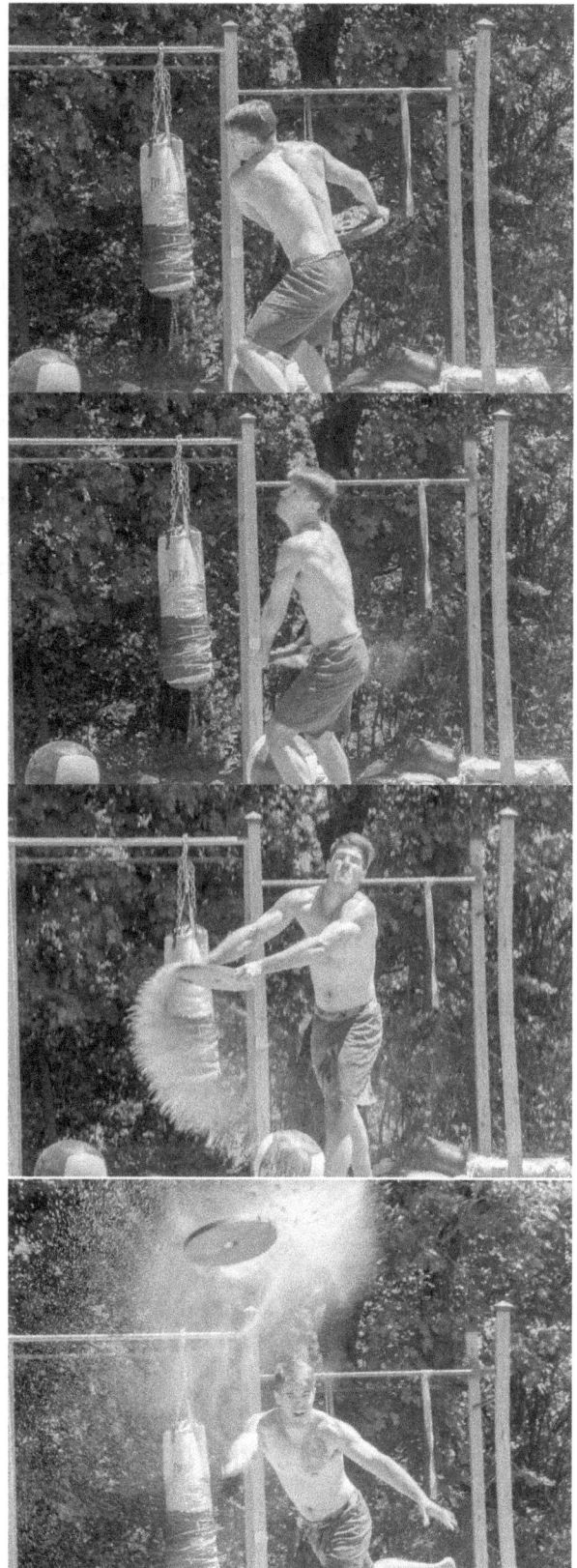

Low Hurdle Hops in the Sand

Classification: Lower Body Power/Quickness

Exercise Prerequisites: Four week familiarization and adaptation to sand training is recommended prior to engaging in high intensity jump training in the sand. You may want to avoid if you have Achilles tendon, knee, hip, low back, ankle, or neck issues.

Movement: Set up 5-10 low (less than 12") hurdles roughly 2-3 feet apart. Standing erect, with feet hip width apart and toes pointing forward or slightly out, jump as high as you can over the hurdle pulling your knees up toward your chest. Once you land, minimize ground contact time and jump as high as you can over the next hurdle, once again pulling your knees toward your chest. Make sure your feet do not kick your butt, instead pulling your knees to your chest so your feet are slightly out in front of your body.

Keys to Movement:

1. Keeping torso erect, jump as high as you can pulling your knees toward your chest.
2. Utilize a countermovement arm swing with each jump.
3. Land properly, minimize ground contact time, and jump again over the next hurdle.
4. Make sure your feet do not kick your butt.

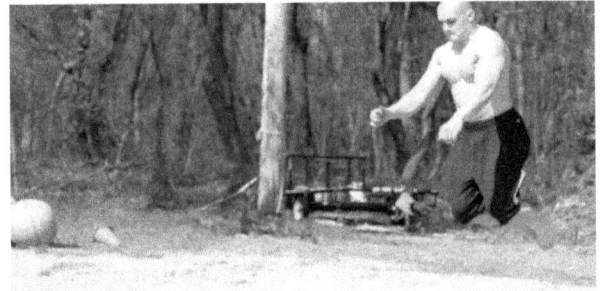

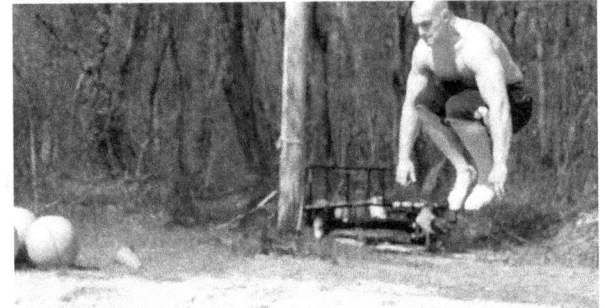

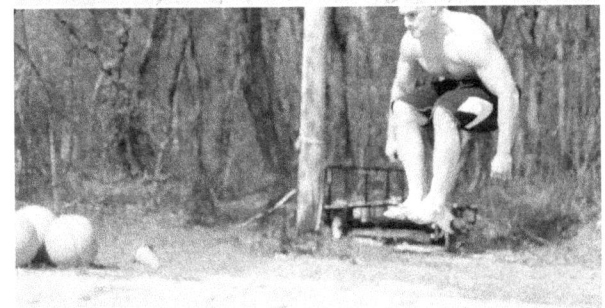

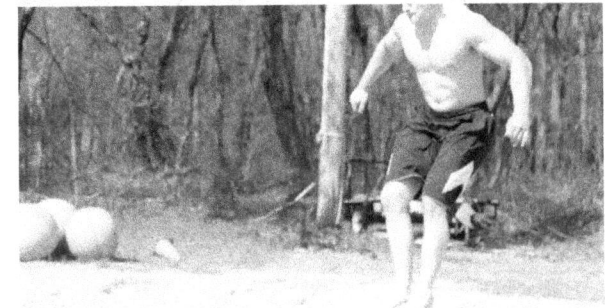

Low Hurdle Lateral Hops in the Sand

Classification: Lateral Movement/Power/Quickness

Exercise Prerequisites: Four week familiarization and adaptation to sand training is recommended prior to engaging in high intensity jump training in the sand. You may want to avoid if you have Achilles tendon, knee, hip, low back, ankle, or neck issues.

Movement: Stand sideways roughly 1-2 feet from a low hurdle (less than 12"). Standing erect, with feet roughly hip width apart and toes pointing forward or slightly out, jump as high as you can laterally over the hurdle pulling your knees up toward your chest. Land with two feet on the other side of the hurdle, minimize ground contact time, then jump laterally back over the hurdle as high as you can, once again pulling your knees toward your chest. Make sure your feet do not kick your butt, instead pulling your knees to your chest so your feet are slightly out in front of your body.

Keys to Movement:

1. Stand sideways next to a low hurdle with feet roughly hip width apart and toes pointing forward.
2. Utilize a countermovement arm swing and jump as high as you can laterally over the hurdle.
3. Land with optimal landing mechanics, minimize ground contact time, and reverse direction jumping back over the hurdle as high as you can.
4. Make sure your feet do not kick your butt.

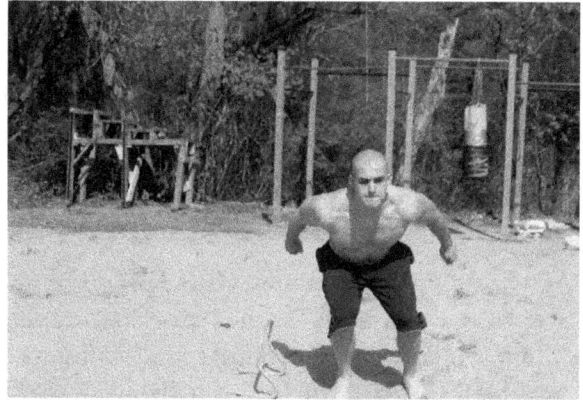

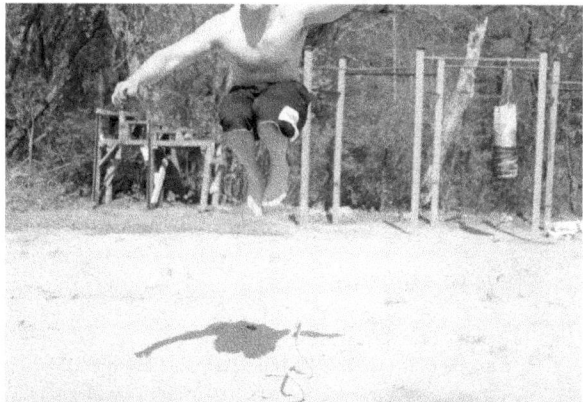

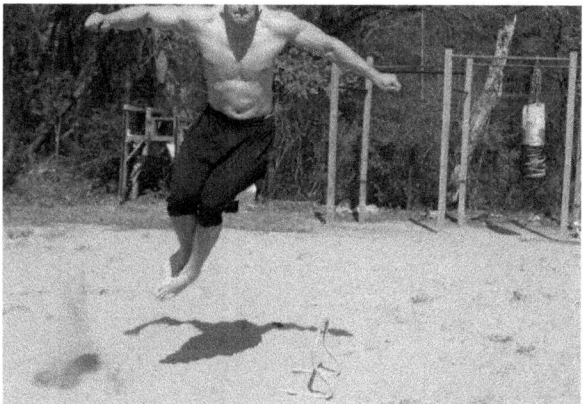

Med Ball Nukem' in the Sand

Classification: Total Body Power and Conditioning

Exercise Prerequisites: Avoid if chronic neck, knee, shoulder or low back pain.

Movement: Set up volleyball net in the sand. Teams of two using a 6-20 lb. medicine ball depending on the experience, strength levels, and injury profiles of the athletes. Throw the ball over the net and the other team must catch the ball. The ball is thrown from where the opposing player catches the ball. Points are awarded each time the ball goes out of bounds, doesn't go over the net, or the opposing team drops the ball.

Keys to Movement:

1. Teams of two are ideal.
2. Anywhere from a 6-20 lb. med ball works well.
3. Throws can be lateral or press. Try to limit overhead or Viking toss throws as catching the ball at these heights can be potentially dangerous.

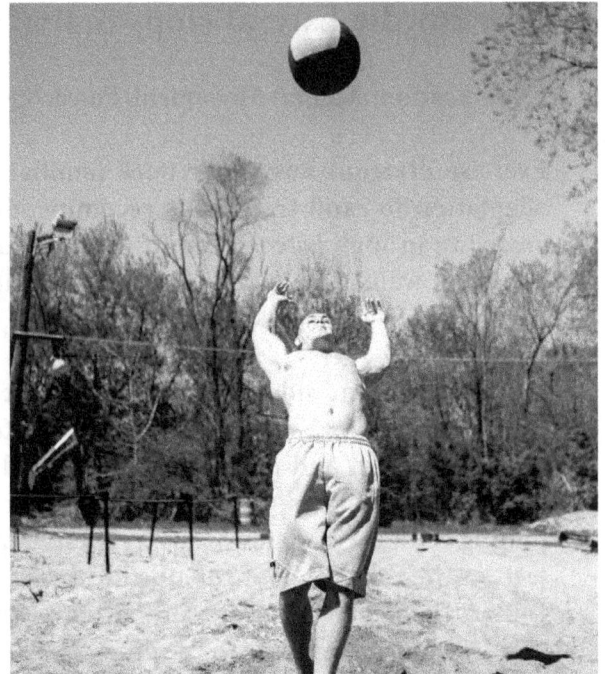

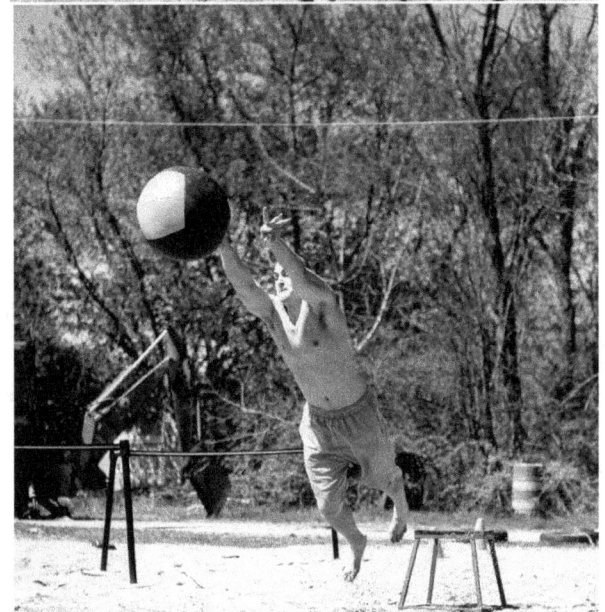

Overhead Keg Carry

Classification: Total Body Strength and Stability

Exercise Prerequisites: Avoid if chronic neck, knee, shoulder or low back pain.

Movement: Begin by placing a keg on its side in front of you. Try to maintain a neutral to lordotic back posture to lift the keg, (though you may need to allow for a kyphotic lifting posture), with feet either wide or close depending on comfort level and body type. Keeping your knees slightly bent, lift the keg to your hips. Once at your hips use triple extension technique similar to that of a mid-thigh/hip power clean to "pop" the keg up to your chest/shoulders. Once the keg is chest/shoulder height, use a "jerk" or push press technique to drive the keg up overhead. Be sure to keep the keg balanced when overhead. Drop the keg either in front of you or behind you if you begin to lose balance. Once stable, walk for predetermined time or distance. Try to maintain extension in shoulders and arms, with rigid upright torso posture throughout.

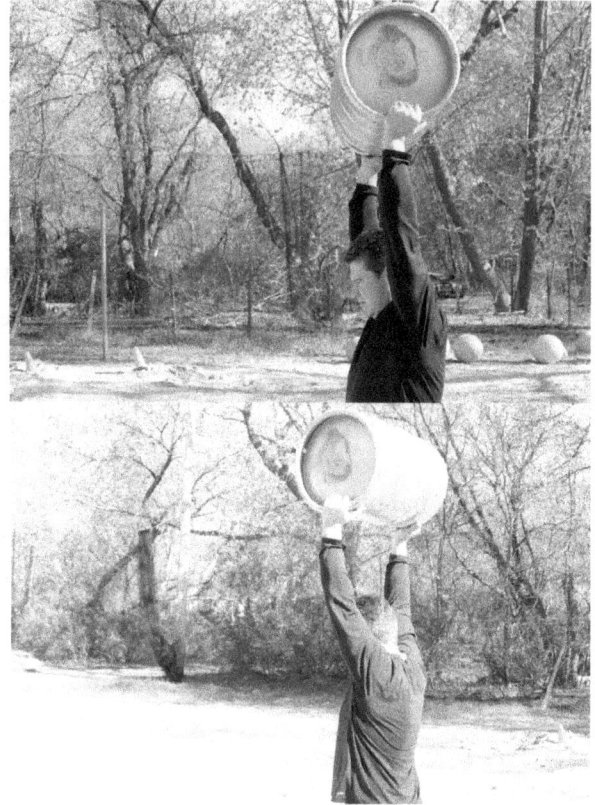

Keys to Movement:

1. Use proper "Clean and Jerk" method to pop the keg up overhead.
2. Keeps shoulders and arms extended to stabilize the keg overhead.
3. Try to maintain rigid upright torso posture.
4. Walk for predetermined time or distance.

Overhead Slosh Stick Carry

Classification: Total Body Strength and Stability

Exercise Prerequisites: Avoid if chronic neck, knee, shoulder or low back pain.

Movement: A slosh stick is a long (generally 6-10 feet) PVC pipe, preferably 2-4" in diameter. These are usually filled half to three quarters with water. To perform the Overhead Slosh Stick Carry, begin by lifting the stick to a jerk position. Once you have "creatively" lifted the stick to this position, jerk it overhead. Be sure to keep the stick balanced and posture rigid. Once stable begin to walk, trying to follow a straight line without allowing the stick to deviate your from course. Drop the stick either in front of you or behind you if you begin to lose balance.

Keys to Movement:

1. Jerk the stick overhead.
2. Keeps shoulders and arms extended to stabilize the stick overhead.
3. Try to maintain rigid upright torso posture.
4. Walk for predetermined time or distance.

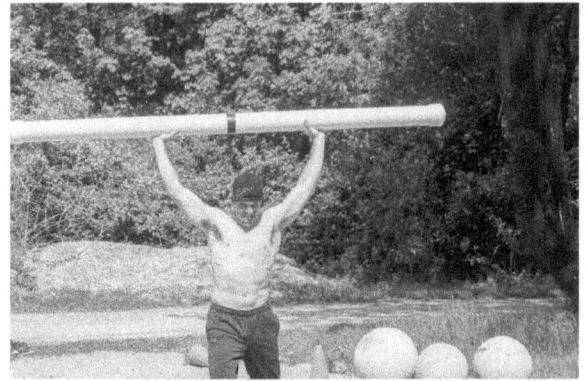

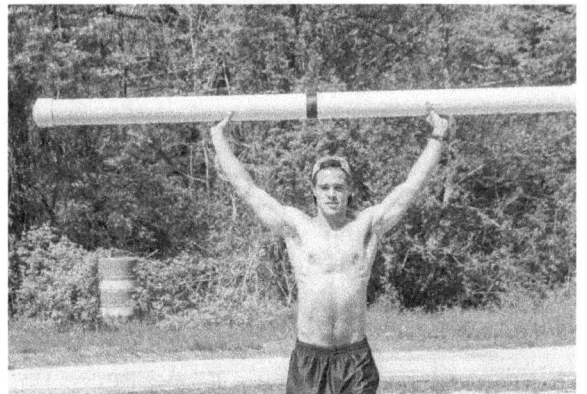

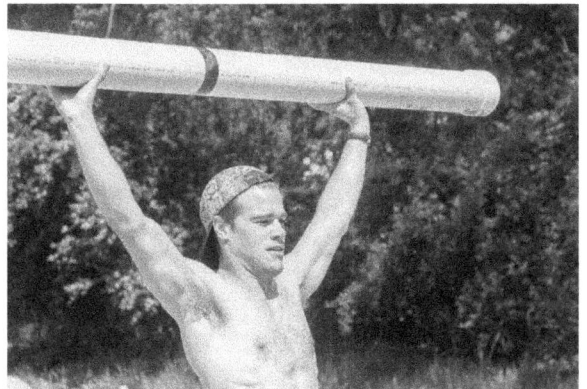

Overhead Walking Lunges in the Sand

Classification: Leg Strength/Total Body Strength and Stability

Exercise Prerequisites: Avoid if you have persistent neck, knee, or low back pain.

Movement: Position body with feet hip width apart, torso in neutral/slightly lordotic posture, with weight plate held in both hands directly overhead (be sure to fully extend shoulder and arms). Maintain upright posture throughout movement. With toes pointing straight ahead, take a large step forward. Lower the hips forward and toward the ground maintaining upright posture with no lean forward. Keeping the back leg as straight as possible, descend until the hamstring comes in contact with the calf on the front leg. It is imperative not to lean forward or allow the front foot heel to come off the ground throughout the movement. As the hamstring comes in the contact with the calf, the knee may cross the toe plane. If the knees are healthy, this can help to strengthen the knee as there is a greater VMO, adductor, hamstring, and gluteal activation with deeper squats and lunges. Once the back knee is 1-2" above the ground initiate the upward/forward drive with the front foot heel, pulling the body forward and up into the original start position without the non-ground contact foot touching the ground until the next step. Keep the plate overhead and torso upright throughout the entire movement. Perform the same for the other leg, driving the knee and lunging forward, performing in a cyclic walking pattern.

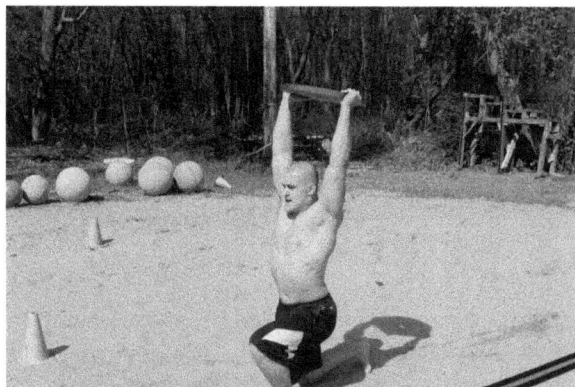

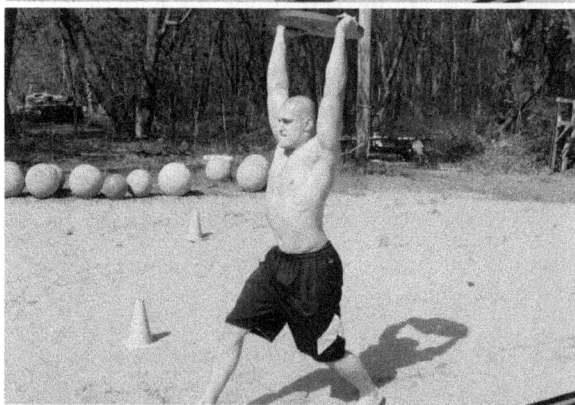

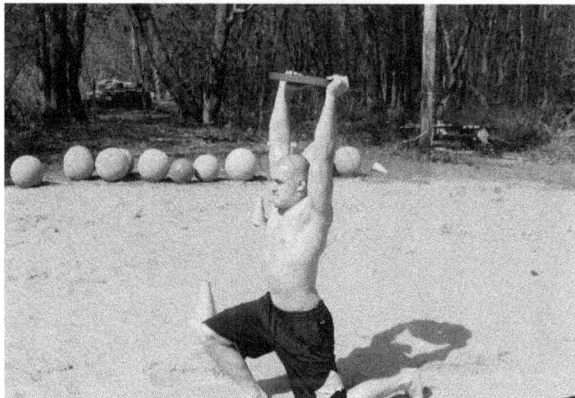

Pogo Jumps in the Sand

Classification: Lower Body Power, Stability, and Conditioning

Exercise Prerequisites: Avoid if chronic knee, shoulder, neck or low back pain.

Movement: Jump as high as you can with minimal bend in the knees and maximal force in the ankles, while keeping your spine in a neutral posture with your shoulder blades pulled slightly back. This is a reactive movement with no pause in between repetitions. As soon as you land on the ground, bounce back up in the air minimizing ground contact time. Do not let the heels touch the ground throughout the set.

Keys to Movement:

1. Jump as high as you can with minimal bend in the knees and torso.
2. Try to minimize ground contact time while maximizing jump height.
3. Do not leg your heels make contact with the sand throughout the movement.

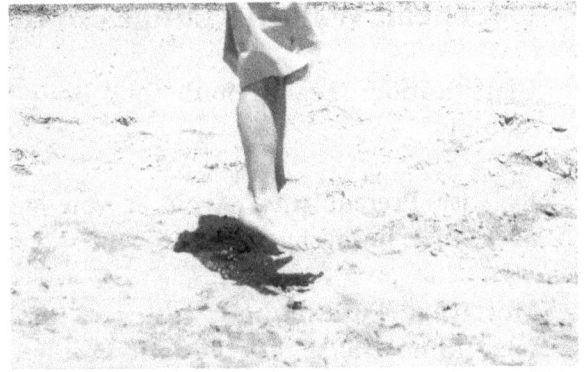

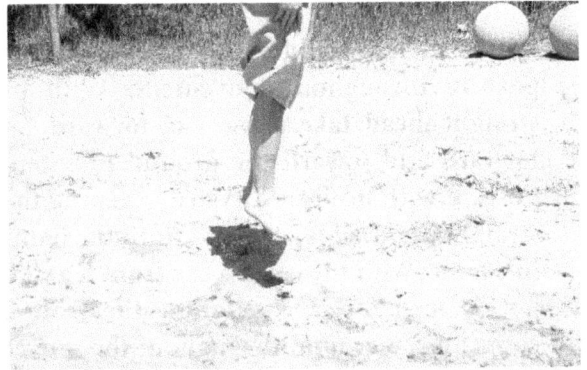

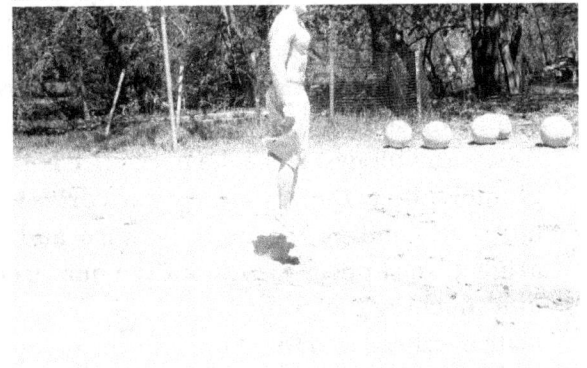

Power Clean from hang above knee to Broad Jump in the Sand Complex

Classification: Total Body Power

Exercise Prerequisites: Avoid if chronic neck, knee, shoulder or low back pain.

Movement: Perform a conventional power clean from mid-thigh to hip hang position on a solid platform near the sandpit. Rest roughly 30 seconds and perform a broad jump in the sand.

Keys to Movement:

1. Utilize proper power clean technique. For more on power clean technique check out our section on Olympic lifts in The In-Season Training Manual. Taking a USAW course or learning Olympic Lifting technique from a USAW certified coach is also recommended.
2. Upon completion of predetermined repetitions of power clean, rest roughly 30 seconds and perform a broad jump in the sand.

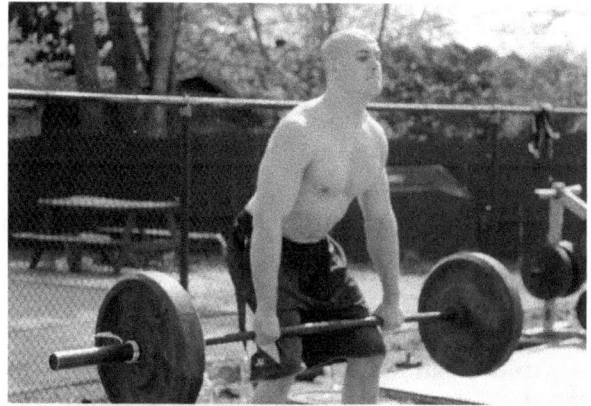

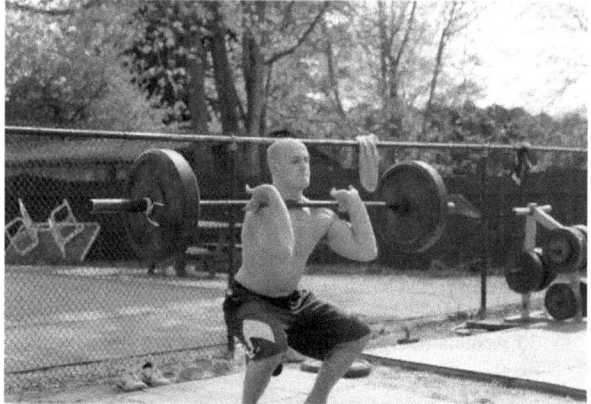

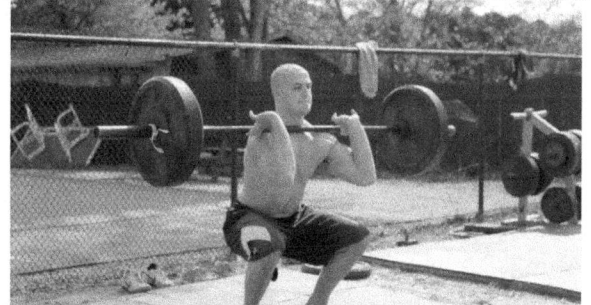

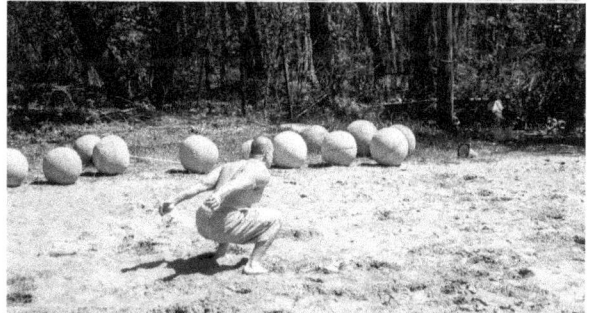

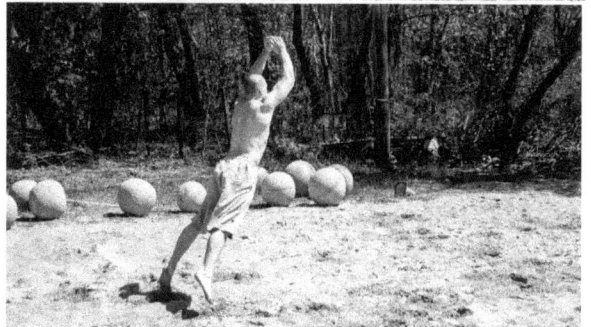

Power Clean from hang above knee to Depth Jump in the Sand Complex

Classification: Total Body Power

Exercise Prerequisites: Avoid if chronic neck, knee, shoulder or low back pain.

Movement: Perform a conventional power clean from mid-thigh to hip hang position on a solid platform near the sandpit. Rest roughly 30 seconds and perform a depth jump (non-plyometric) in the sand.

Keys to Movement:

1. Utilize proper power clean technique. For more on power clean technique check out our section on Olympic lifts in The In-Season Training Manual. Taking a USAW course or learning Olympic Weightlifting technique from a USAW certified coach is also recommended.
2. Upon completion of predetermined repetitions of power clean, rest roughly 30 seconds and perform predetermined repetitions of non-true plyometric depth jumps in the sand.

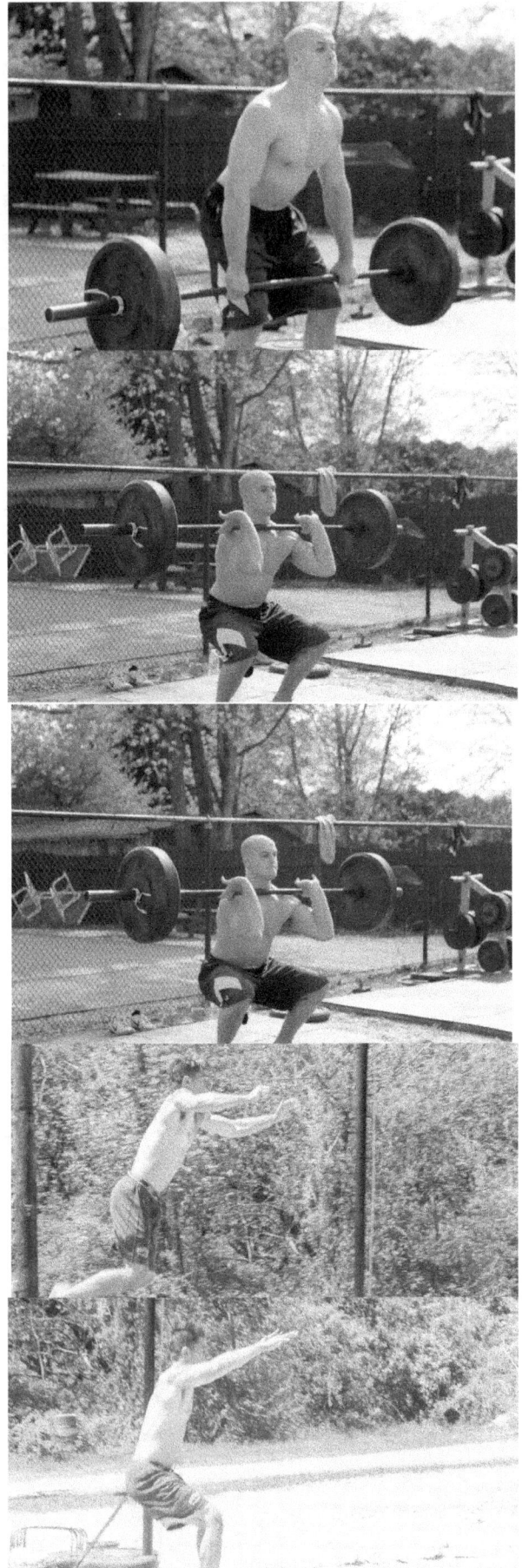

Power Clean from hang above knee to Overhead Throw in the Sand Complex

Classification: Total Body Power

Exercise Prerequisites: Avoid if chronic neck, knee, shoulder or low back pain.

Movement: Perform a conventional power clean from mid-thigh to hip hang position on a solid platform near the sandpit. Rest roughly 30 seconds and perform an overhead throw with implement of your choice in the sand.

Keys to Movement:

1. Utilize proper power clean technique. For more on power clean technique check out our section on Olympic lifts in The In-Season Training Manual. Taking a USAW course or learning Olympic Weightlifting technique from a USAW certified coach is also recommended.

2. Upon completion of predetermined repetitions of power clean, rest roughly 30 seconds and perform an overhead throw with the implement of your choice in the sand.

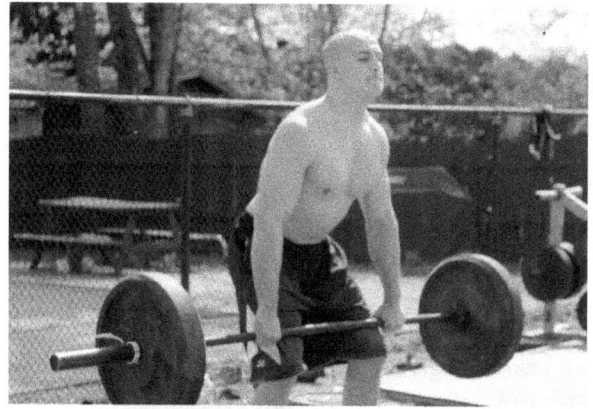

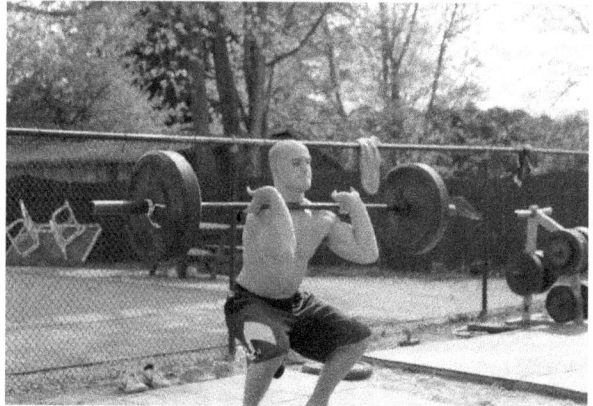

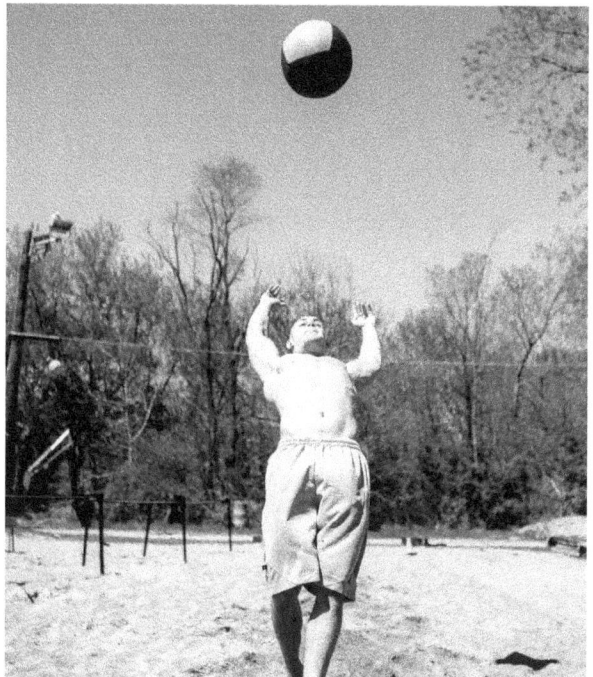

Power Clean from hang above knee to Resisted Sled Sprint in the Sand Complex

Classification: Total Body Power and Acceleration

Exercise Prerequisites: Avoid if chronic neck, knee, shoulder or low back pain.

Movement: Perform a conventional power clean from mid-thigh to hip hang position on a solid platform near the sandpit. Rest roughly 30 seconds and perform a light resisted sled sprint in the sand.

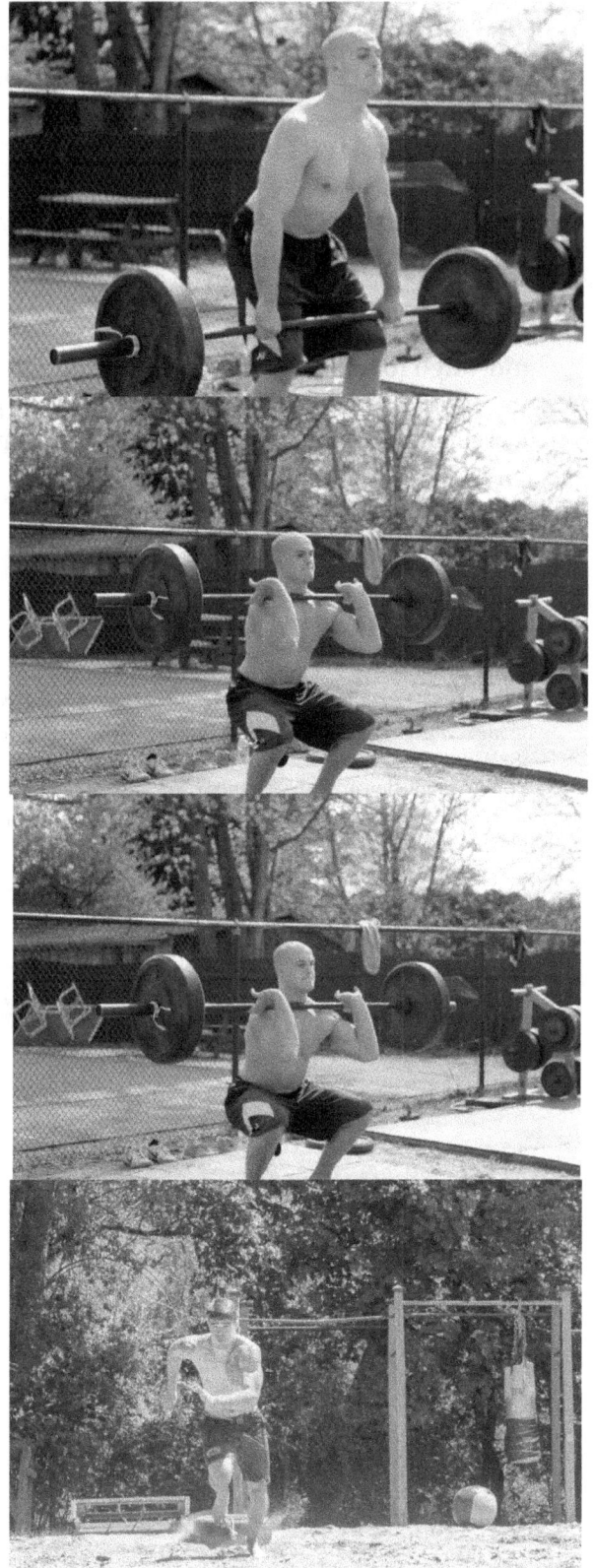

Keys to Movement:

1. Utilize proper power clean technique. For more on power clean technique check out our section on Olympic lifts in The In-Season Training Manual. Taking a USAW course or learning Olympic Weightlifting technique from a USAW certified coach is also recommended.

2. Upon completion of predetermined repetitions of power clean, rest roughly 30 seconds and perform a light resisted sprint in the sand.

Power Clean from hang above knee to Sprint in the Sand Complex

Classification: Total Body Power and Acceleration

Exercise Prerequisites: Avoid if chronic neck, knee, shoulder or low back pain.

Movement: Perform a conventional power clean from mid-thigh to hip hang position on a solid platform near the sandpit. Rest roughly 30 seconds and perform a maximal short sprint in the sand.

Keys to Movement:

1. Utilize proper power clean technique. For more on power clean technique check out our section on Olympic lifts in The In-Season Training Manual. Taking a USAW course or learning Olympic Weightlifting technique from a USAW certified coach is also recommended.
2. Upon completion of predetermined repetitions of power clean, rest roughly 30 seconds and perform a maximal effort short distance sprint in the sand.

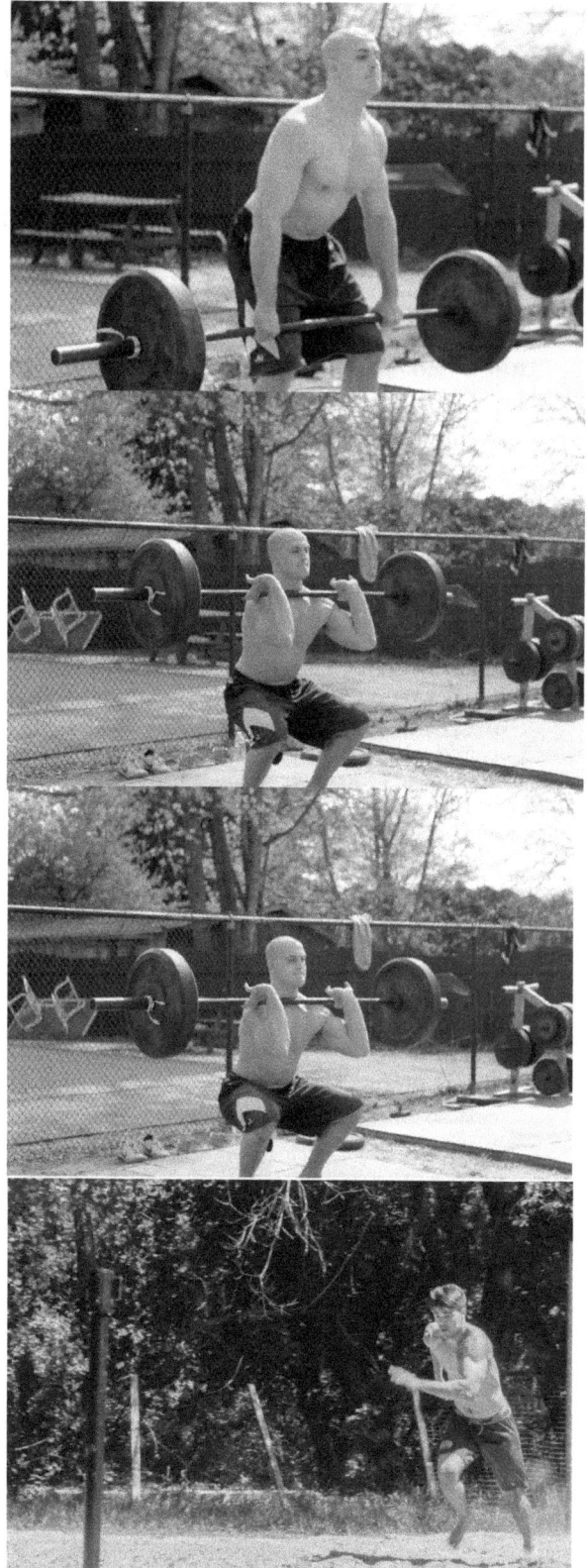

Power Clean from hang above knee to Vertical Jump in the Sand Complex

Classification: Total Body Power

Exercise Prerequisites: Avoid if chronic neck, knee, shoulder or low back pain.

Movement: Perform a conventional power clean from mid-thigh to hip hang position on a solid platform near the sandpit. Rest roughly 30 seconds and perform a vertical jump in the sand.

Keys to Movement:

1. Utilize proper power clean technique. For more on power clean technique check out our section on Olympic lifts in The In-Season Training Manual. Taking a USAW course or learning Olympic Weightlifting technique from a USAW certified coach is also recommended.

2. Upon completion of predetermined repetitions of power clean, rest roughly 30 seconds and perform predetermined repetitions of vertical jumps in the sand

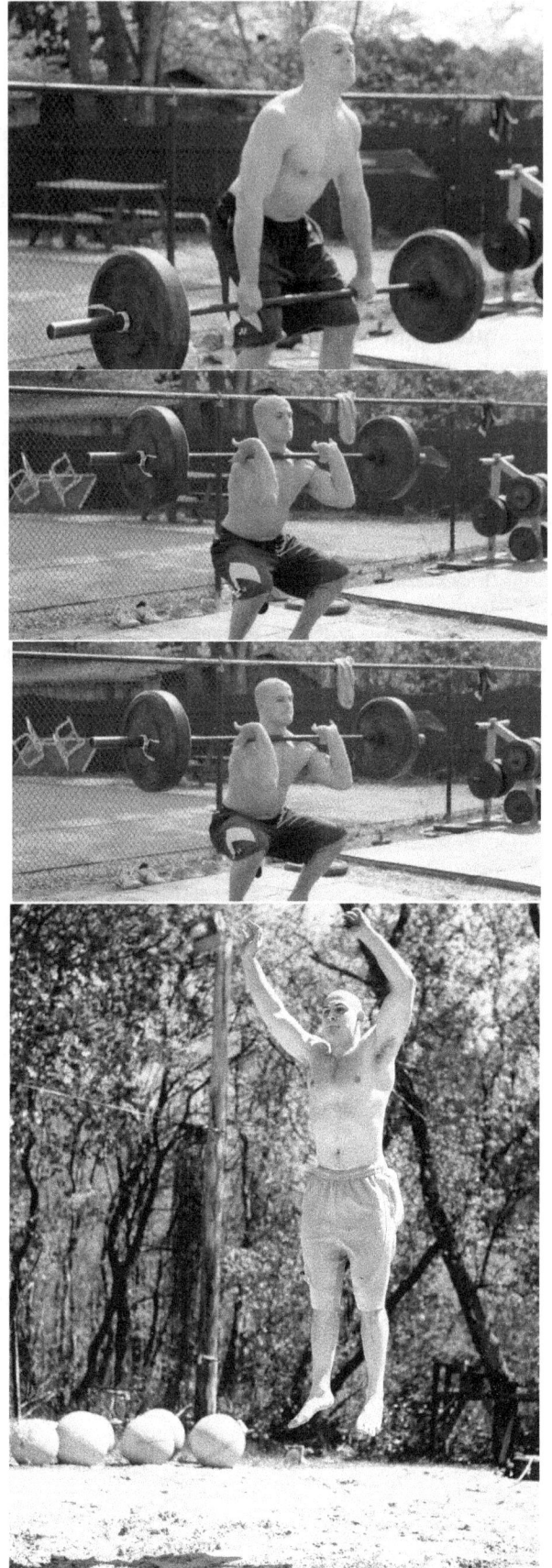

Power Skips in the Sand

Classification: Speed/Acceleration/Stability

Exercise Prerequisites: Avoid if chronic neck, knee, shoulder or low back pain.

Movement: Skip as high as you can, kicking your opposite knee up as high as you are comfortable. Minimize ground contact time while maintaining stable upright posture. Utilize optimal arm swing mechanics.

Keys to Movement:

1. Maintain stable upright posture.
2. Minimize ground contact time while skipping as high as you can.

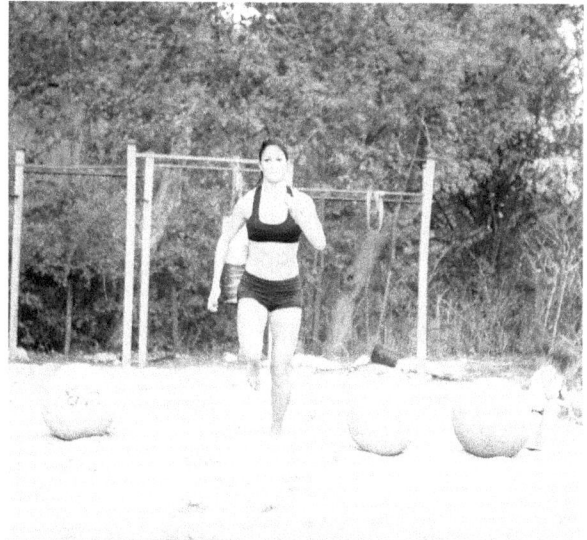

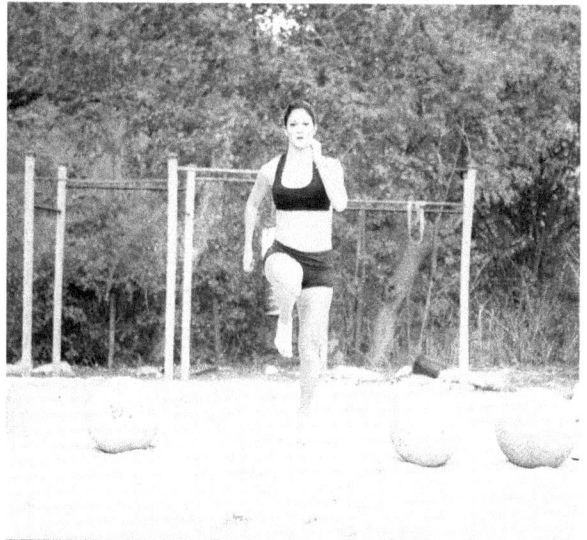

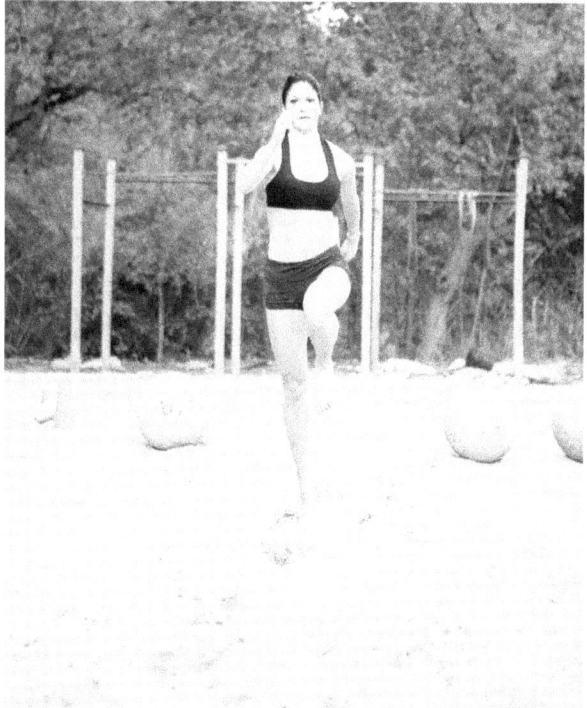

Quick Feet Forward Agility Ladder Drill in the Sand

Classification: Warm-up/Quickness

Exercise Prerequisites: Avoid if chronic neck, knee, shoulder or low back pain.

Movement: Stand at one end of the agility ladder. Keeping knees low, quick step each foot into each rung. Maintain stable upright posture and minimize ground contact times.

Keys to Movement:

1. Minimize ground contact time.
2. Maintain stable upright posture.

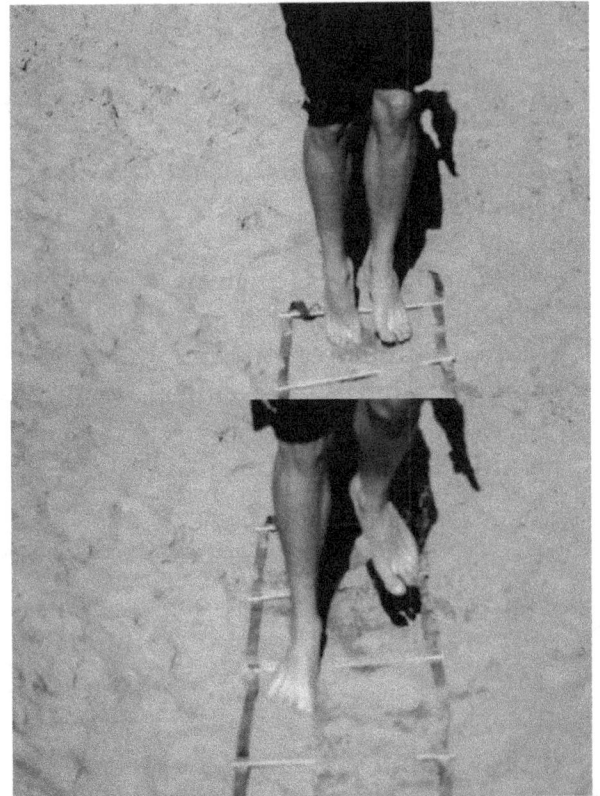

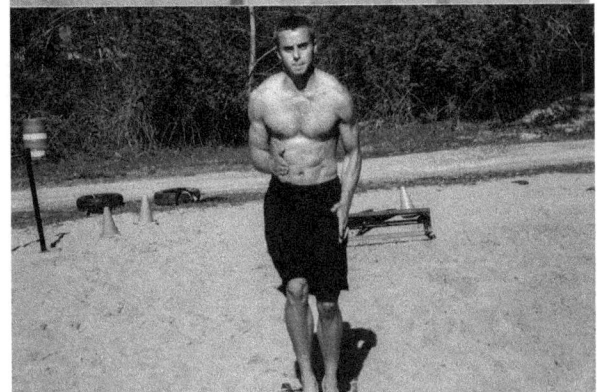

Sand Low Crawl

Classification: Total Body Conditioning

Exercise Prerequisites: Avoid if chronic neck, knee, shoulder or low back pain.

Movement: Position strings, ropes, or low hurdles as low crawl obstacles. Start with chest, hips, thighs, feet, and elbows on the sand. Keeping your head low, shoot one arm out straight in front of you. Keeping chest, hips, knees and feet in contact with the ground, follow with the same side knee driving upward out to the side. Then switch sides, pulling with one side while driving forward with the other arm, followed by other knee. Be sure to keep your chest and hips as low as possible during the duration of the crawl.

Keys to Movement:

1. Try to keep chest, hips, knees, and feet in contact with the sand.
2. Drive one arm out in front then follow with the same side knee driving forward and out to your side. .
3. Switch sides and pull with one side while driving forward with the other.

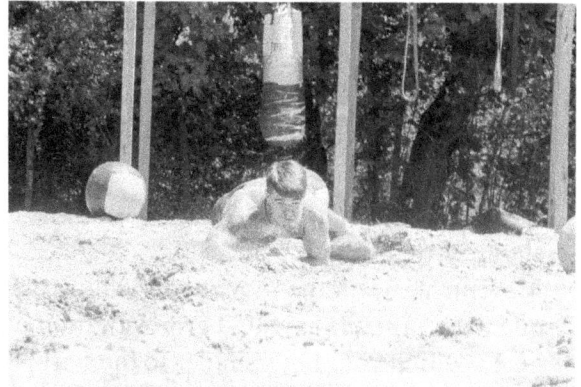
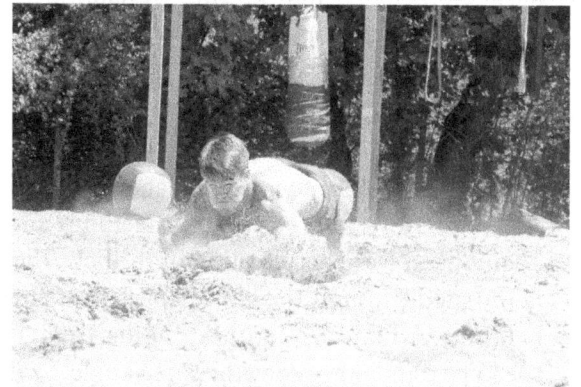
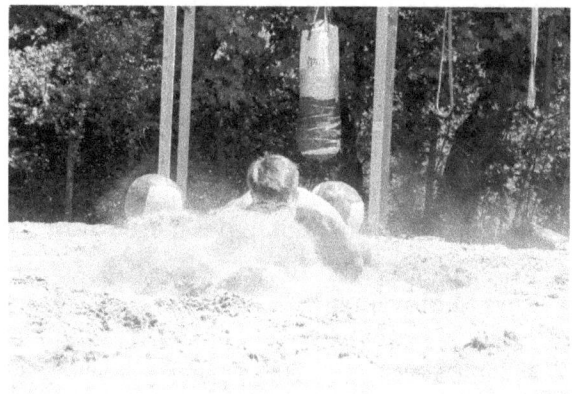

Single Arm Trap-3 Overhead Kettlebell Throw

Classification: Total Body Power and Trap-3 Strengthening

Exercise Prerequisites: Avoid if chronic neck, knee, shoulder or low back pain.

Movement: Begin the movement holding the kettlebell in one hand utilizing a neutral grip with thumb away. From here position your body similar to the start position of the basic kettlebell swing. Be sure to bend at the knees and waist when positioning into the start position. This ensures the muscle tension is created in the glutes and hamstrings, rather than the low back.

Swing the bell between the legs, about knee to shin height. At the point of full tension on the glutes and hamstrings begin the upward acceleration of the bell. The upward pull is initiated through the glutes and hamstrings. Swing the bell outward and upward, extending the hips, extending the knees, and increasing the torso angle. Swing the bell in an arcing fashion above your head with the angle between your arm and neck at roughly 45 degrees. Be sure to keep the neutral grip throughout. At the top of the movement, release the bell upward and backward, aiming for roughly a 45 degree trajectory. A good tip is to keep eyes focused on straight ahead with neutral head posture to ensure optimal recruitment of trap-3 musculature.

Keys to Movement:

1. Start in optimal kettlebell swing position holding kettlebell in one hand with neutral grip, thumb away.
2. Swing the bell once or twice to gain momentum for throw.
3. Swing the bell downward/inward until optimal tension on glutes and hamstrings, and then reverse direction driving the kettlebell upward and outward.
4. Try to ensure roughly a 45 degree angle between arm and neck at top of range of motion or release point.
5. Release the bell once you reach extension.

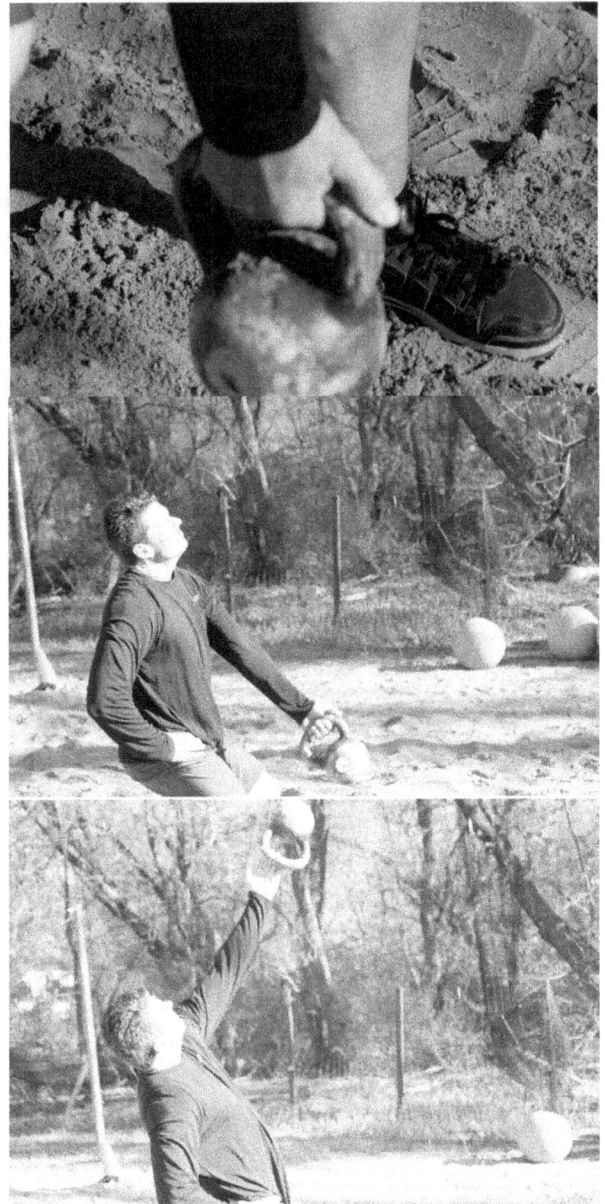

Single Arm Overhead Kettlebell Throw

Classification: Total Body Power

Exercise Prerequisites: Avoid if chronic neck, knee, shoulder or low back pain.

Movement: Begin the movement holding the kettlebell in one hand and positioning the body similar to the start position of the basic kettlebell swing. Be sure to bend at the knees and waist when positioning into the start position. This ensures the muscle tension is created in the glutes and hamstrings, rather than the low back.
Grab the kettlebell with one hand, palm facing you. Swing the bell between the legs, about knee to shin height. At the point of full tension on the glutes and hamstrings begin the upward acceleration of the bell. The upward pull is initiated through the glutes and hamstrings. Swing the bell outward and upward, extending the hips, extending the knees, increasing the torso angle. Swing the bell in an arcing fashion above your head, keeping the arm extended, ending up on the toes. At the top of the movement, release the bell upward and backward, aiming for roughly a 45 degree trajectory. A good tip is to follow the path of the bell with your eyes to ensure optimal mechanics.

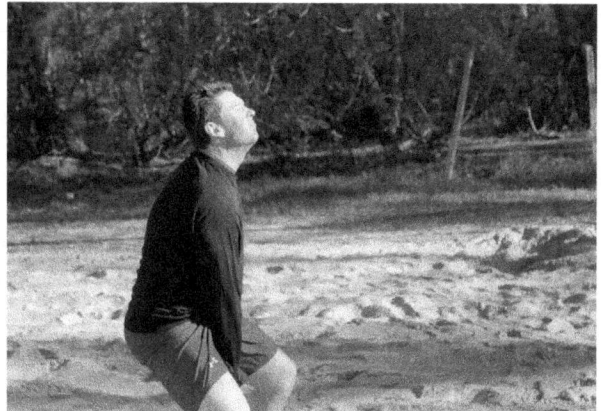

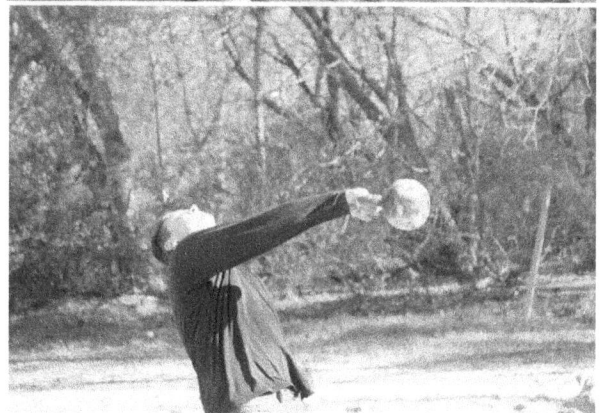

Keys to Movement:

1. Start in optimal kettlebell swing position.
2. Swing the bell once or twice to gain momentum for throw.
3. Swing the bell downward/inward until optimal tension on glutes and hamstrings, and then reverse direction driving the kettlebell upward and outward.
4. Release the bell once you reach extension of the hips, knees, ankles, and shoulder.
5. Aim for a 45 degree trajectory behind you to ensure safety.
6. Keep your eyes on the bell to ensure optimal movement mechanics and safety.

Single Leg Low Hurdle Hops in the Sand

Classification: Lower Body Stability and Quickness

Exercise Prerequisites: Four week familiarization and adaptation to sand training is recommended prior to engaging in high intensity jump training in the sand. You may want to avoid if you have Achilles tendon, knee, hip, low back, ankle, or neck issues.

Movement: Set up 5-10 low (less than 12") hurdles roughly 2-3 feet apart. Standing erect on one foot with toes pointing forward, over the hurdle maintaining control of torso and non-working leg. Once you land, minimize ground contact time and jump over the next hurdle. Make sure your foot does not kick your butt, instead pulling your knee upward.

Keys to Movement:

1. Keeping torso erect, jump maintaining control of torso and non-working leg.
2. Feel free to utilize a countermovement arm swing with each jump.
3. Land properly, minimize ground contact time, and jump again over the next hurdle.
4. Make sure your feet do not kick your butt.

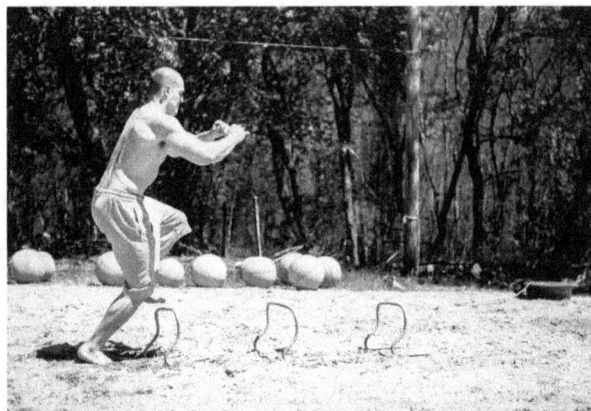

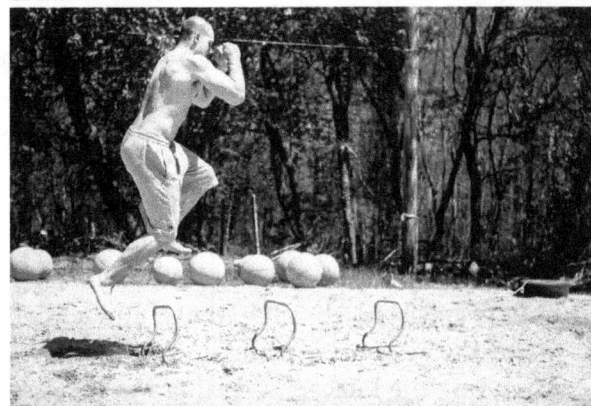

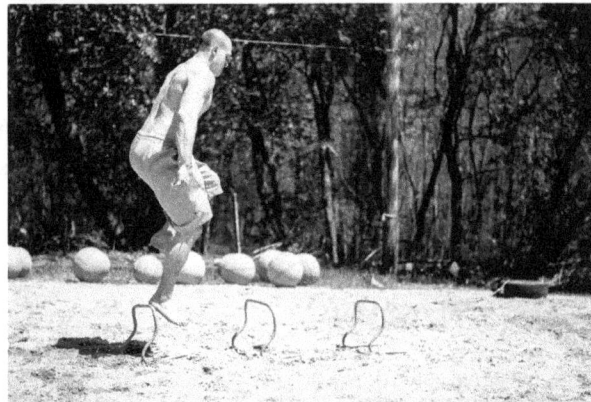

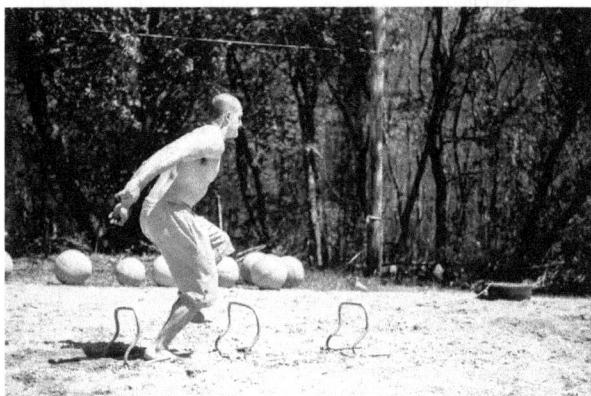

Skater Hops in the Sand

Classification: Acceleration/Power and Stability

Exercise Prerequisites: Four week familiarization and adaptation to sand training is recommended prior to engaging in high intensity jump training in the sand. You may want to avoid if you have Achilles tendon, knee, hip, low back, ankle, or neck issues.

Movement: Start on one leg with roughly 20-40 degree bend at knee and neutral to lordotic posture. Kick opposite leg behind you, flex the hip, and lean your torso out past your knee. Swing your arms downward and behind. At the point of optimal tension in the glutes and hamstrings, swing your arms upward and outward, jumping upward and at an angle outward. You do not want to jump straight out or directly to the side. Land with optimal landing mechanics on the opposite leg, keeping torso posture rigid. Perform same mechanics for other leg.

Keys to Movement:

1. Stand on one leg, keeping torso posture neutral/lordotic, and perform countermovement swing downward.
2. At point of optimal tension in glutes and hamstrings, swing arms upward and outward and jump at roughly a 45 degree angle outward onto the opposite leg.
3. Land with optimal landing mechanics and perform again with other leg.

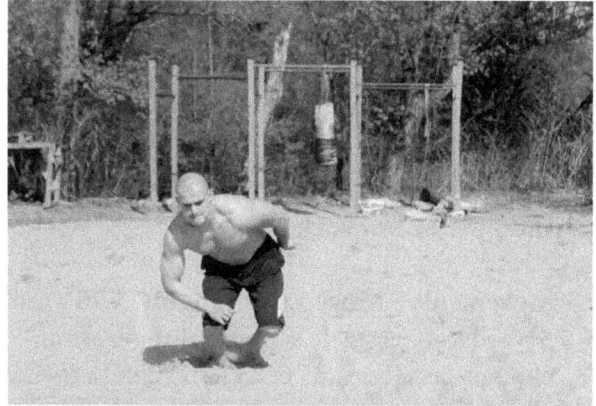

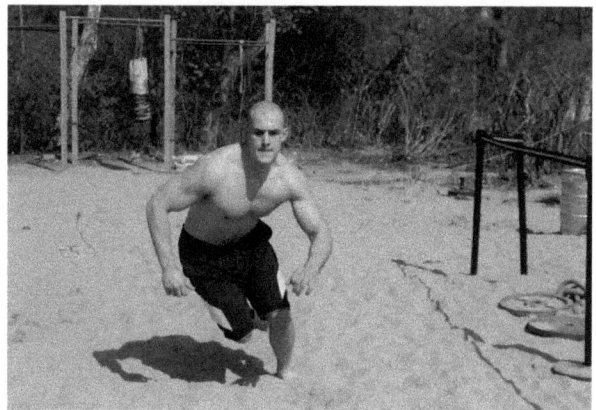

Slalom Agility Sprint in the Sand

Classification: Agility and Conditioning

Exercise Prerequisites: Avoid if chronic neck, knee, shoulder or low back pain.

Movement: Set up cones roughly 5-10 yards wide and 5 yards apart in a slalom configuration. After each change, accelerate as fast as you can to the next cone.

Keys to Movement:

1. Accelerate as fast as you can from one cone to the next.
2. Utilize optimal deceleration and change of direction mechanics.

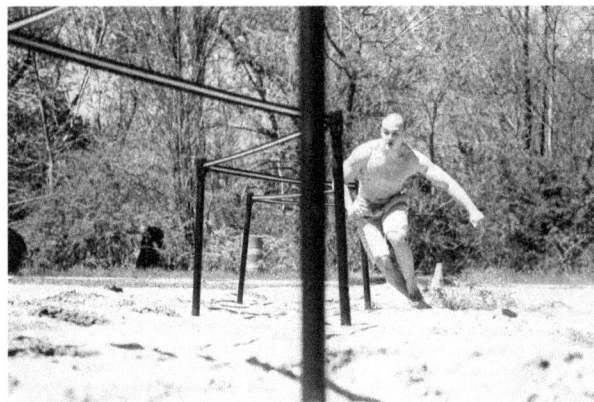

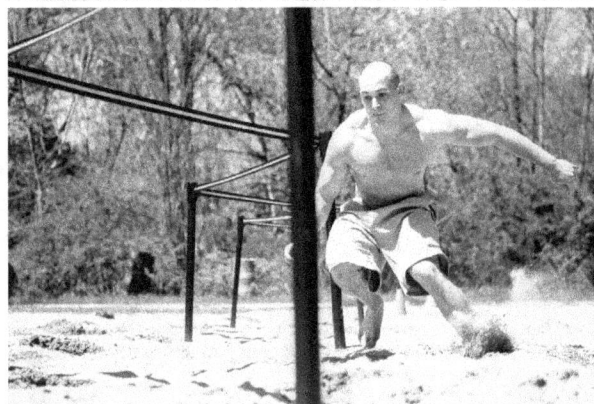

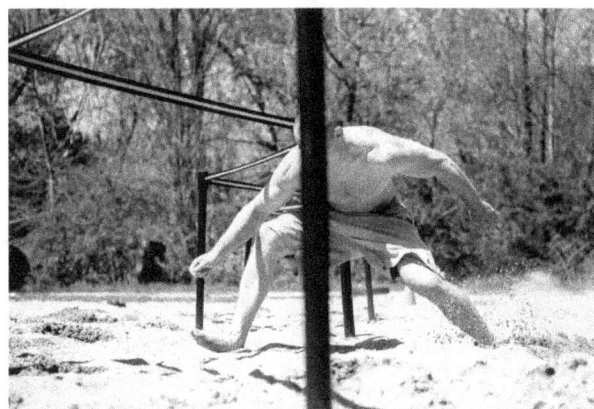

Sledgehammer Sand Hits

Classification: Total Body General Physical Preparation

Exercise Prerequisites: Avoid if chronic knee, shoulder, neck or low back pain.

Movement: Starting at the side, swing the sledghammer ovehead and hit into the sand. Options include alternating sides, same side hits, walking forward hits, walking backward hits, and lateral walking hits.

Keys to Movement:

1. Start holding sledghammer at your side.
2. Swing up and around and hit the gound as hard as you can.
3. Alternate sides or perform on ssame side.

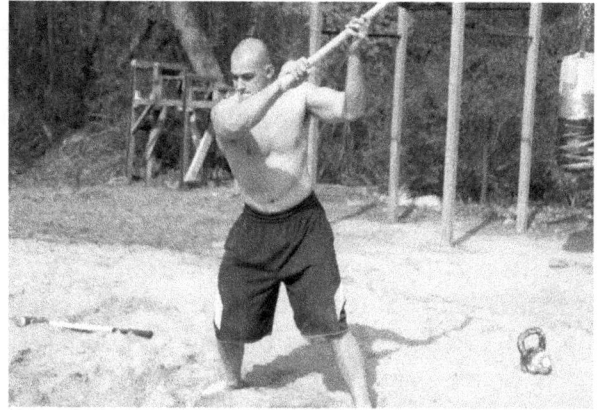

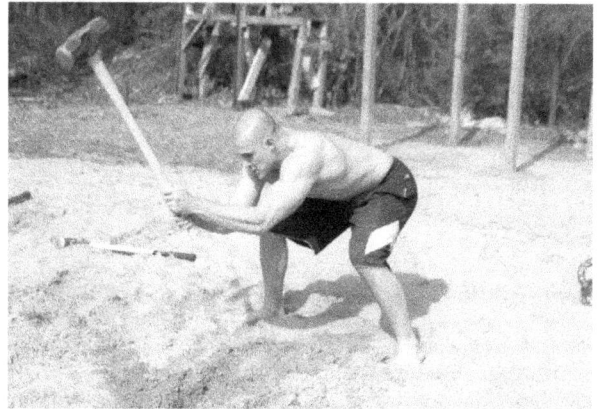

Split Jumps in the Sand

Classification: Unilateral Stability and Power

Exercise Prerequisites: Avoid if chronic knee, shoulder, neck or low back pain.

Movement: Start in an optimal split squat position with roughly 90 plus degree angle at the front knee and back leg comfortably extended behind you. Perform a downward arm swing to generate elastic stretch. Immediately change direction and swings arms outward and upward, jumping as high as you can into the air. Scissor kick your legs so that you land with legs in opposite positions. Immediately swing back downward and perform again.

Keys to Movement:

1. Start in optimal split squat position.
2. Swing arms powerfully downward until optimal stretch in front leg glutes and hamstrings.
3. Rapidly change direction swinging arms outward and upward, propelling your body into the air. .
4. Scissor kick in the air and alternate lead and trail legs.

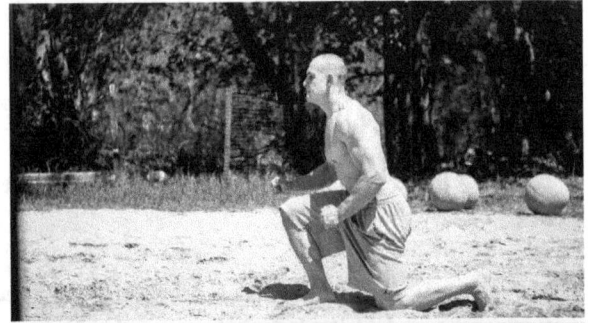

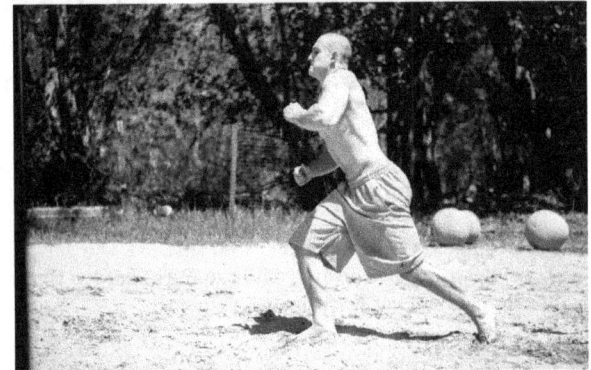

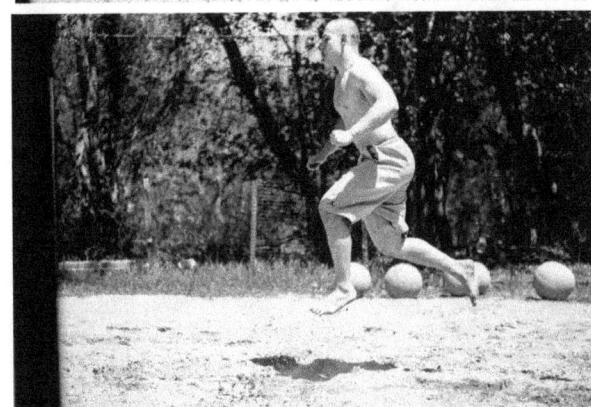

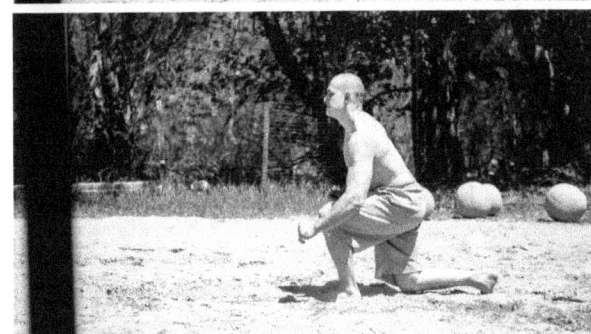

Squat Jumps in the Sand

Classification: Lower Body Power/Conditioning

Exercise Prerequisites: Avoid if chronic knee, shoulder, neck or low back pain.

Movement: With feet roughly hip to shoulder width apart, squat downward using optimal body squat mechanics. Squat to roughly thighs parallel to the sand, trying to keep torso as upright as possible. Extend hips, knees, and ankles, jumping as high as you can into the air. Upon landing drop into thighs parallel squat position and perform again for desired repetitions.

Keys to Movement:
1. Start with feet roughly hip to shoulder width apart.
2. Squat down to roughly thighs parallel to sand while keeping your torso upright.
3. Powerfully extend hips, knees, and ankles, propelling your body straight up into the air.
4. Upon landing, immediately drop back down into squat position and perform for desired repetitions.

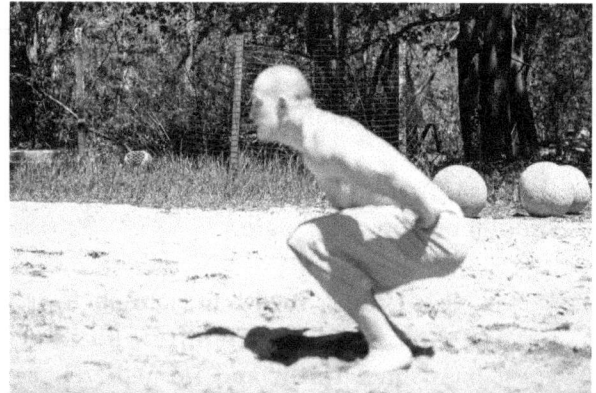

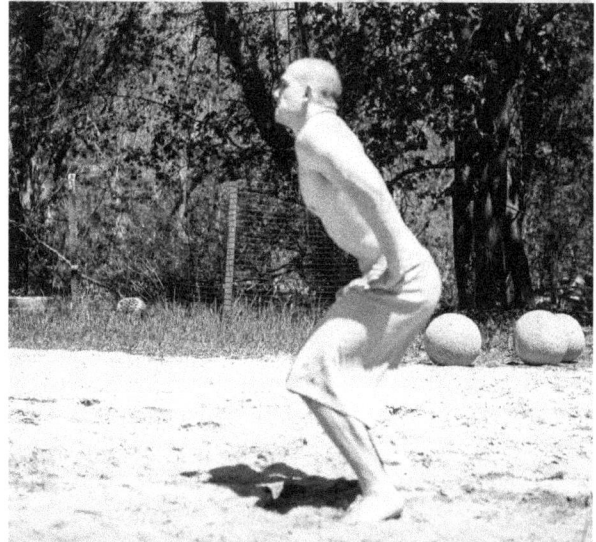

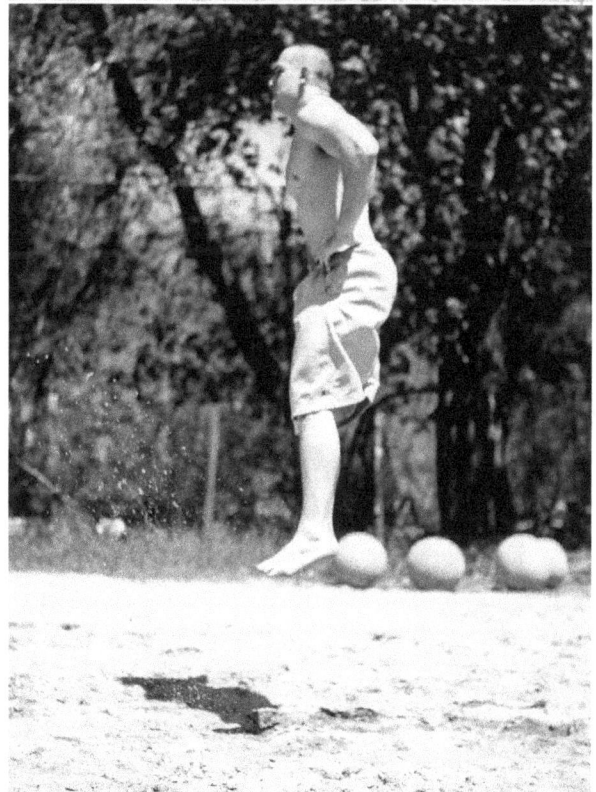

Squat Throw To Sprint in the Sand

Classification: Total Body Power/Acceleration

Exercise Prerequisites: Avoid if chronic neck, knee, shoulder or low back pain.

Movement: Hold a med ball, kettlebell or implement of your choice in chest pass throw position. Perform a chest pass squat throw and immediately sprint a predetermined distance.

Keys to Movement:

1. Squat throw and immediately sprint once you release the ball.

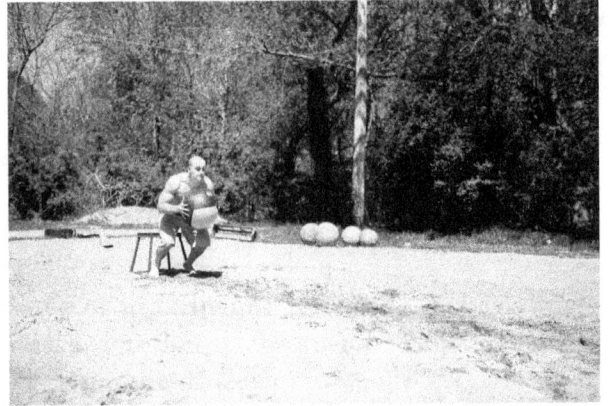

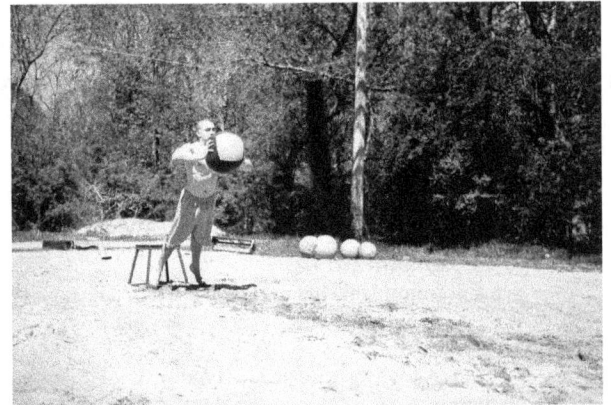

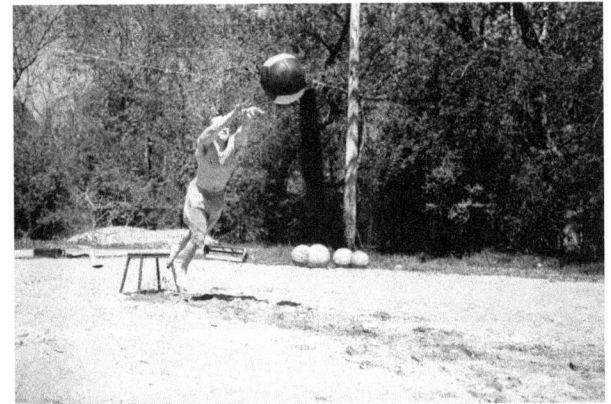

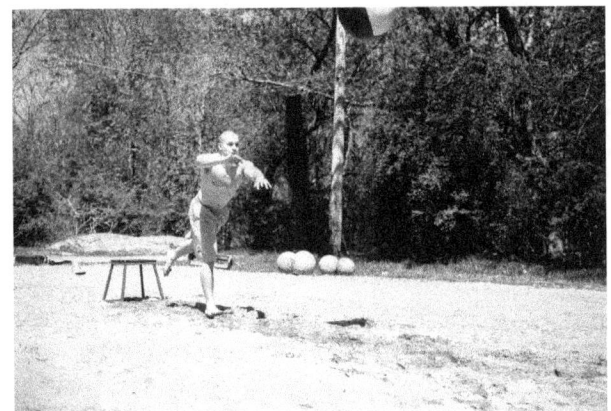

Standing Triple Jump in the Sand

Classification: Lower Body Power and Acceleration

Exercise Prerequisites: Avoid if chronic knee, shoulder, neck or low back pain.

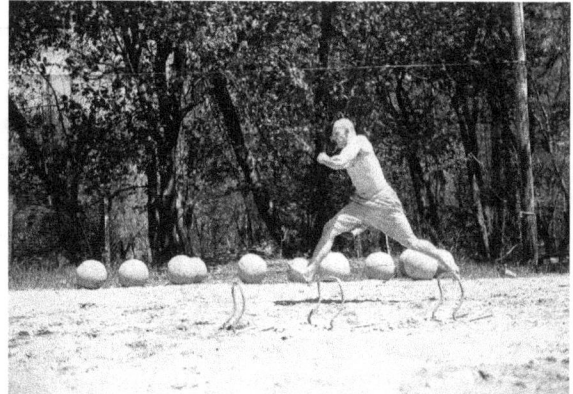

Movement: First set up as you would a broad jump. Perform broad jump countermovement and jump out and land on one leg. Properly absorb the impact with the landing leg, then immediately swing the arms and jump as far as possible off that leg and onto the other leg. From here, single leg jump one more time as far as you can, this time landing on two legs. The idea is to cover as much ground as possible with the 3 jumps, keeping the momentum moving forward, and absorbing the impact of each landing while minimizing ground contact time.

Keys to Movement:

1. Start on two feet and jump out onto one leg.
2. Then jump as far as you can off that leg onto the other leg.
3. From here, single leg jump one more time as far as you can, landing on two legs.
4. Try to cover as much distance as you can in three jumps.

Step Forward Lunges in the Sand

Classification: Lower Body Strength and Stability
Exercise Prerequisites: Avoid if you have persistent neck, knee, or low back pain.
Movement: Position body with feet hip width apart, torso in neutral/slightly lordotic posture, with dumbbells held at your sides or barbell across the shoulders or in font squat rack position. Maintain upright posture throughout movement. With toes pointing straight ahead, take a large step forward. Lower the hips forward and toward the ground maintaining upright posture with no lean forward. Keeping the back leg as straight as possible, descend until the hamstring comes in contact with the calf on the front leg. It is imperative not to lean forward or allow the front foot heel to come off the ground throughout the movement. As the hamstring comes in the contact with the calf, the knee may cross the toe plane. If the knees are healthy, this can help to strengthen the knee as there is a greater VMO, adductor, hamstring, and gluteal activation with deeper squats and lunges. Once the back knee is 1-2" above the ground initiate the backward movement through the ball of the front foot by driving the shoulders back to the start position with no change in posture. Perform all reps on one leg, and then perform on the opposite leg.

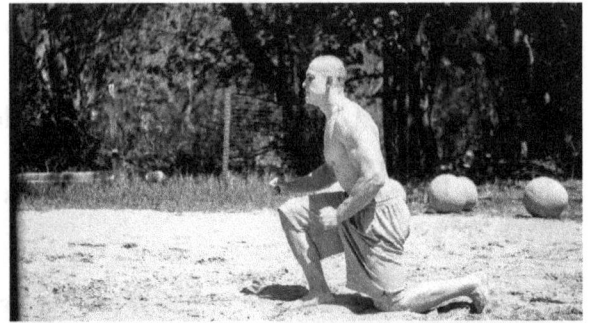

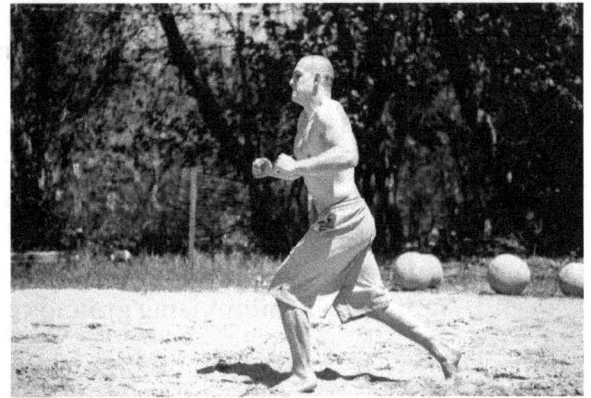

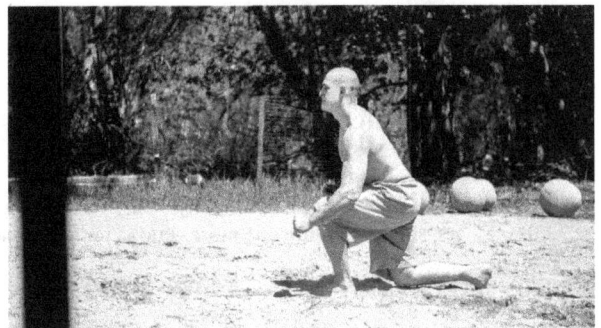

Suitcase Carry

Classification: Total Body Strength and Stability

Exercise Prerequisites: Avoid if chronic neck, knee, shoulder or low back pain.

Movement: Similar to a farmer carry but you will be carrying only one implement rather than two. This is a great exercise to strengthen unilateral imbalances about the low back, hips, and core. Begin by placing the implement of your choice by your side. This may include farmer carry hands, kettlebells, dumbbells, water buckets, etc. Holding neutral to lordotic back posture, with feet either slightly staggered or parallel to each other, and knees bent, place hand on implement handle, Lift using proper deadlift technique. Once stable begin walking, focusing on keeping torso upright, chest high, and shoulders tense. Creating intra-abdominal pressure may also help in keeping the torso rigid and upright. Try not to lean too far away from the resisted side.

Keys to Movement:

1. Lift implement with one arm with proper deadlift technique.
2. Maintain intra-abdominal pressure to stabilize rigid posture.
3. Keep chest high and shoulders tense to maintain posture.
4. Walk for predetermined time or distance.

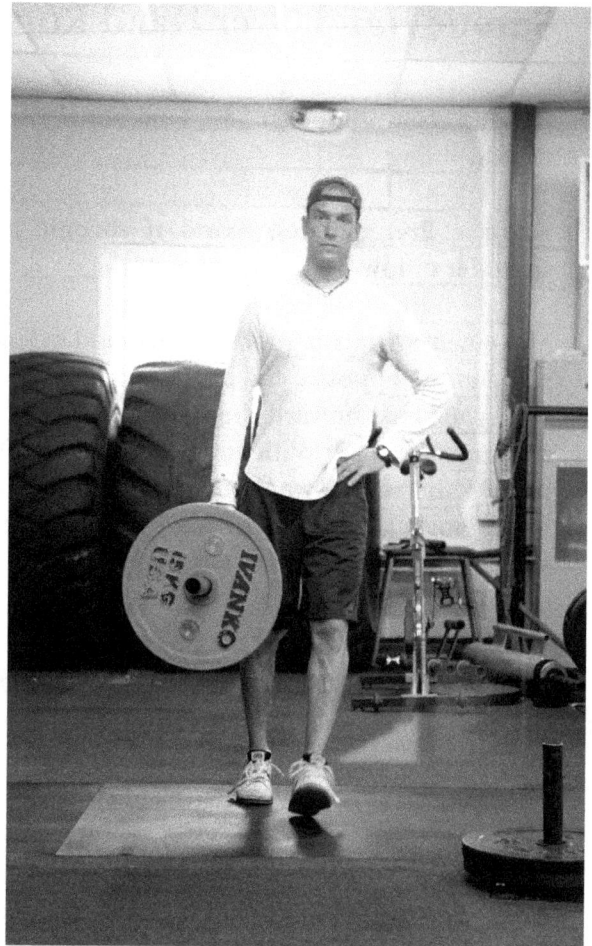

Supine Hand Over Hand Rope Pull

Classification: Upper Body Functional Strength and Conditioning

Exercise Prerequisites: Avoid if chronic neck, knee, shoulder or low back pain.

Movement: Attach a rope to a sled and extend it. Sit or stand at the opposite end of the rope. Lay on your back with your head toward the sled. Reach over your head and grab the rope. With one hand over the other, begin pulling the rope toward you, keeping the elbows tight to the body, alternating hands. Variations may include short pulls, longer pulls, two-handed pulls, pullovers, or triceps pressdown pulls.

Keys to Movement:

1. Safety needs to be paramount. If you have back, shoulder, neck, or elbow issues you may want to forego this exercise.
2. If healthy, feel free to experiment with the different variations of this exercise.

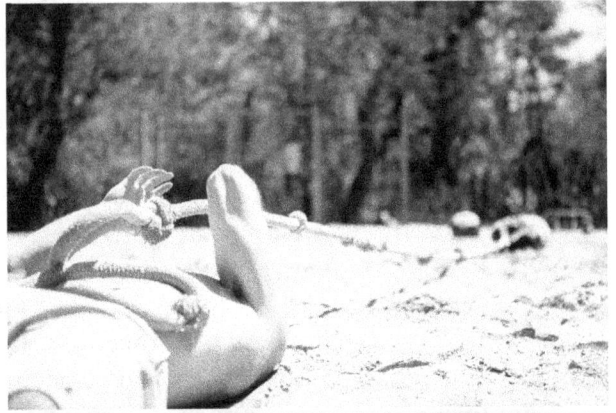

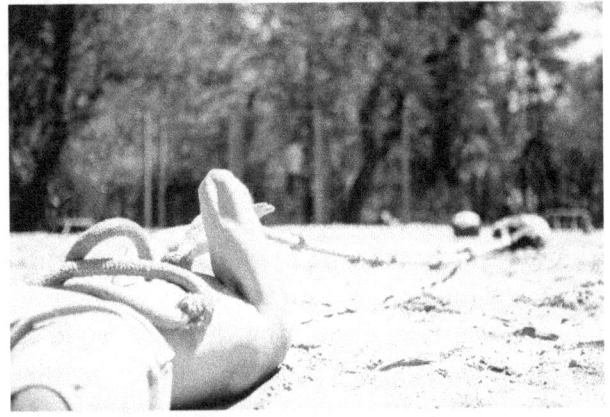

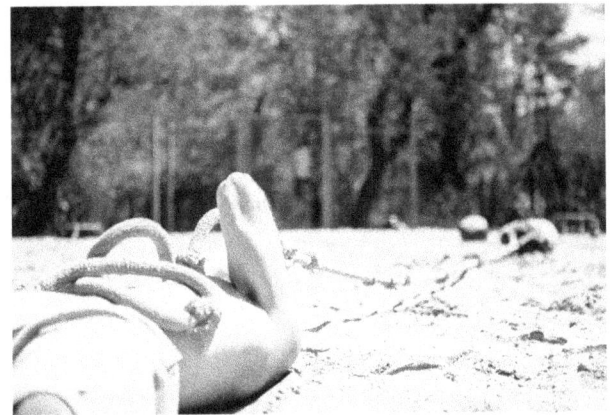

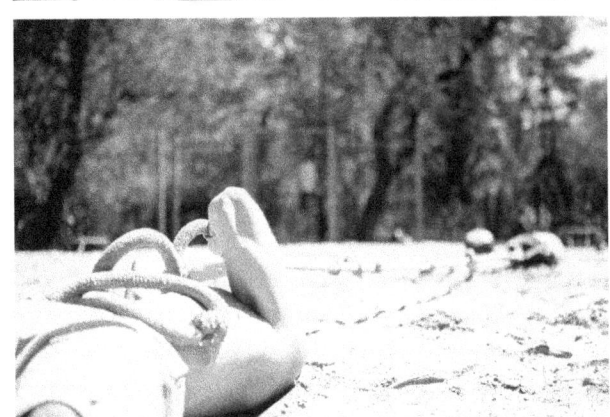

Supine Abdominal Exercises in the Sand

Classification: Torso Flexor and Core Strengthening

Exercise Prerequisites: Avoid if chronic neck, knee, shoulder or low back pain.

Movement: Choose any supine abdominal exercises and perform on the unstable uneven sand surface. Focus on breathing patterns for maximal contraction of abdominal musculature.

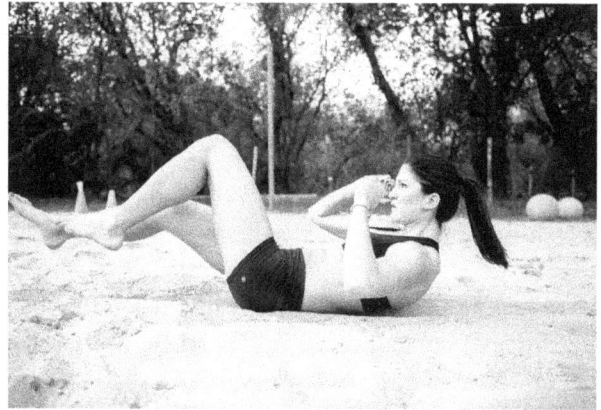

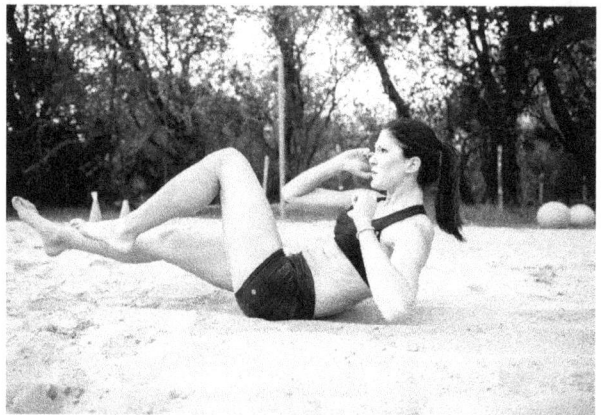

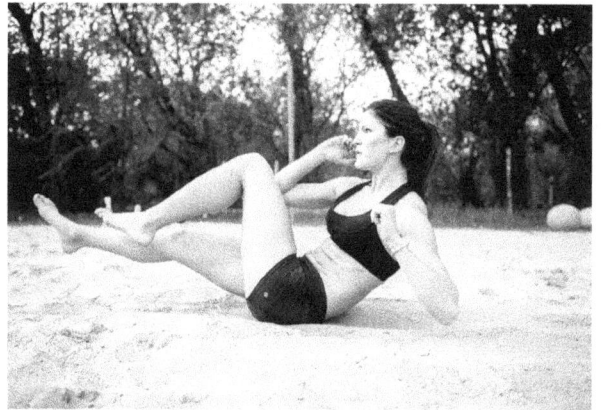

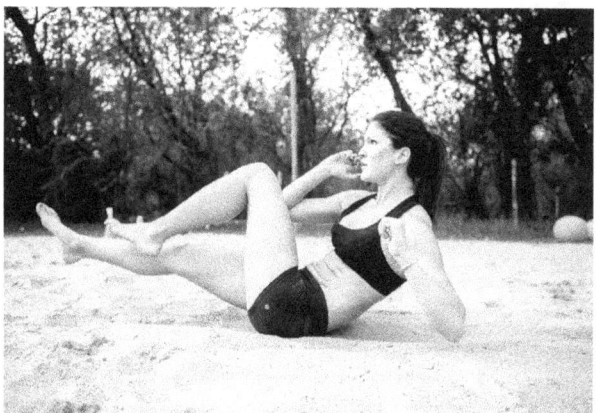

T Drill in the Sand

Classification: Agility

Exercise Prerequisites: Avoid if chronic neck, knee, shoulder or low back pain.

Movement: Set up 4 cones in the shape of a T. The two vertical cones are 10 yards, while the horizontal cones are 5 yards apart from the top vertical cone. Start at the bottom of the T. Sprint 10 yards, side shuffle left 5 yards, side shuffle right 10 yards, side shuffle back to the middle cone, then backpedal back to start.

Keys to Movement:

1. Perform as fast as you can.

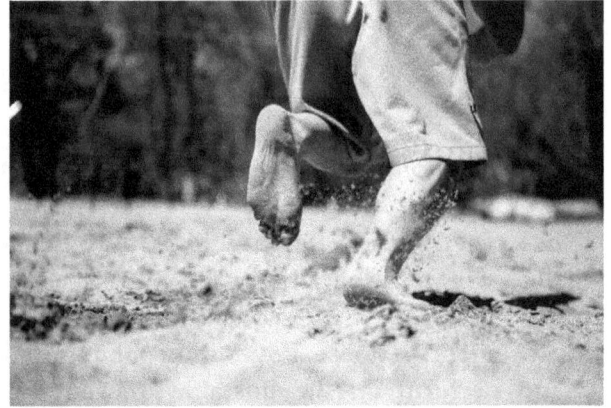

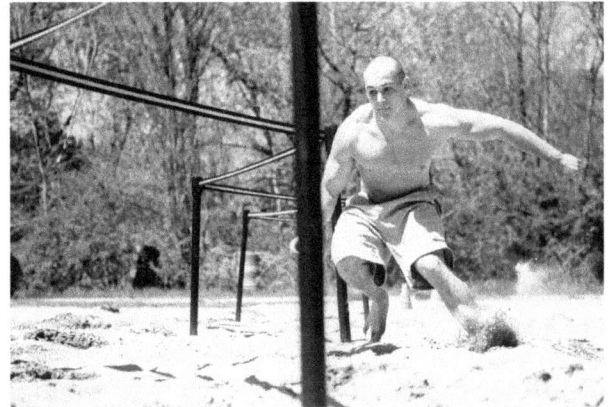

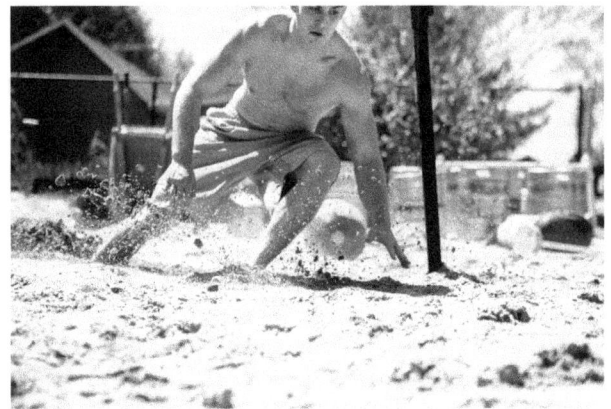

Two Hand Atlas Stone Pull

Classification: Total Body Functional Strength and Conditioning

Exercise Prerequisites: Avoid if chronic neck, knee, shoulder or low back pain.

Movement: Similar to the Hand Over Hand Atlas Stone Pull, but you will pull with both arms at the same time to get the stone rolling. Be sure to keep your feet wide and shuffle your feet as you roll the stone.

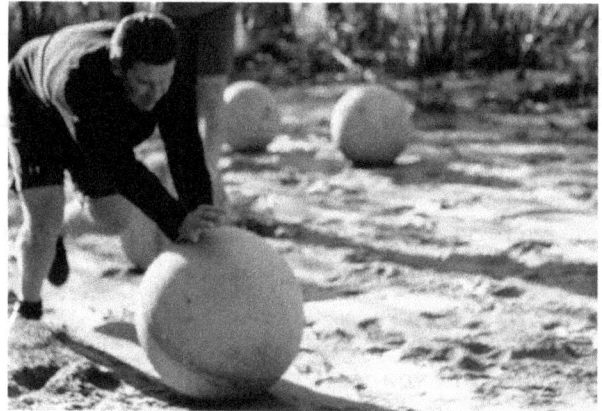

Keys to Movement:

1. Start with two hands on atlas stone with knees bent and torso parallel to the ground.
2. Extend both arms pushing the stone forward.
3. Either shuffle the feet or extend both legs as you drive the stone.
4. Maintain torso as parallel as possible to the ground.
5. Quickly shuffle feet to keep the ball moving forward.
6. Aim for quality of movement first, then try to increase speed or weight of the stone.

Two Hand Atlas Stone Push

Classification: Total Body Functional Strength and Conditioning

Exercise Prerequisites: Avoid if chronic neck, knee, shoulder or low back pain.

Movement: Similar to the Hand Over Hand Atlas Stone Push, but you will extend both arms at the same time to push the stone forward. You can either shuffle your feet and reset with each push or extend both legs as you extend your arms similar to the movement of the Hammer Strength Jammer.

Keys to Movement:

1. Start with two hands on atlas stone with knees bent and torso parallel to the ground.
2. Extend both arms pushing the stone forward.
3. Either shuffle the feet or extend both legs as you drive the stone.
4. Maintain torso as parallel as possible to the ground.
5. Quickly shuffle feet to keep the ball moving forward.
6. Aim for quality of movement first, then try to increase speed or weight of the stone.

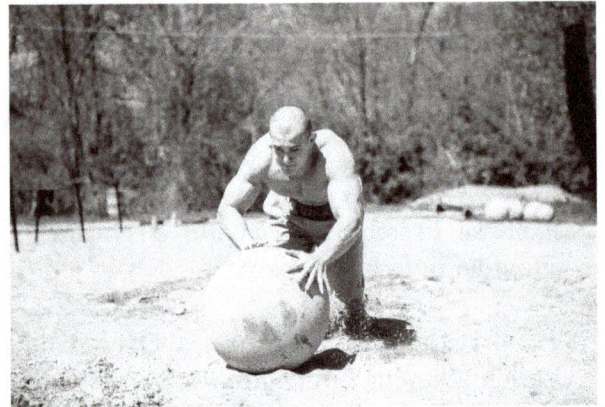

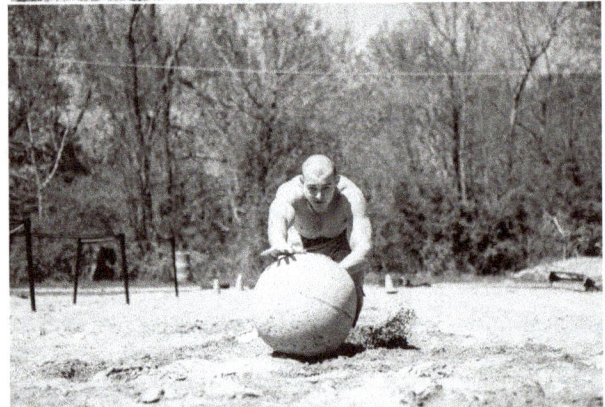

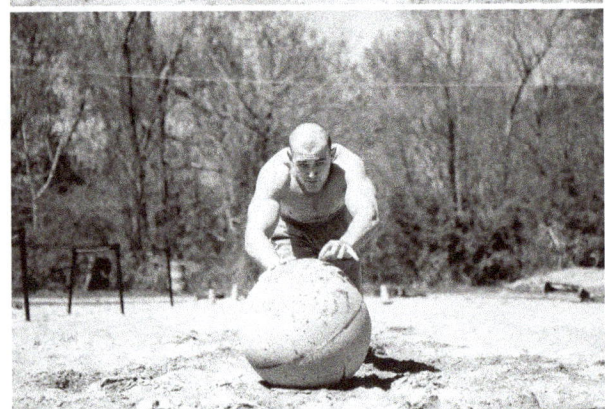

Two Hand Overhead Throw

Classification: Total Body Power

Exercise Prerequisites: Avoid if chronic neck, knee, shoulder or low back pain.

Movement: One of the best parts about training in a sandpit is that you can throw training implements such as kettlebells without risk of damage or breaking. Begin the movement by positioning the body similar to the start position of the kettlebell swing. Be sure to bend at the knees and waist when positioning into the start position. This ensures the muscle tension is created in the glutes and hamstrings, rather than the low back.
Grab the kettlebell with two hands, palms facing you. Swing the bell between the legs, about shin height. At the point of full tension on the glutes and hamstrings begin the upward acceleration of the bell. The upward pull is initiated through the glutes and hamstrings. Swing the bell outward and upward, extending the hips, extending the knees, increasing the torso angle. Swing the bell in an arcing fashion above your head, keeping the arms extended, ending up on the toes. At the top of the movement, release the bell upward and backward, aiming for roughly a 45 degree trajectory. A good tip is to follow the path of the bell with your eyes to ensure optimal mechanics.

Keys to Movement:

1. Start in optimal kettlebell swing position.
2. Swing the bell once or twice to gain momentum for throw.
3. Swing the bell downward/inward until optimal tension on glutes and hamstrings, and then reverse direction driving the kettlebell upward and outward.
4. Release the bell once you reach extension of the hips, knees, ankles, and shoulders.
5. Aim for a 45 degree trajectory behind you to ensure safety.
6. Keep your eyes on the bell to ensure optimal movement mechanics and safety.

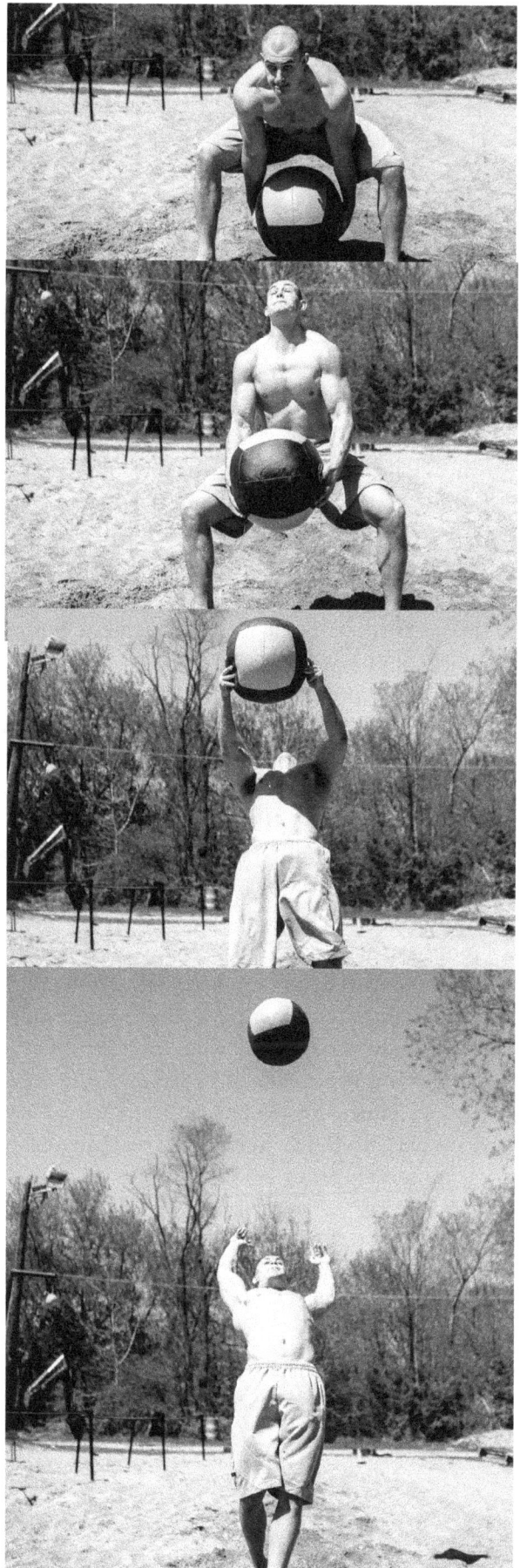

Vertical Jump in the Sand

Classification: Total Body Power

Exercise Prerequisites: Four week familiarization and adaptation to sand training is recommended prior to engaging in high intensity jump training in the sand. You may want to avoid if you have Achilles tendon, knee, hip, low back, ankle, or neck issues.

Movement: The faster you perform the countermovement, the further you will jump. It is Newton's Law which states "for every action, there is an equal and opposite reaction". Picture a tennis ball bouncing against the floor. If you just drop the ball it may rebound upward only 3-4 feet. The reaction is equal to the action. Whereas if you throw the ball with maximal force against the floor the ball will rebound much further. For countermovement jumps, the body works in the manner.

Begin by positioning your feet roughly hip width apart, with knees and toes pointing straight ahead, with shoulders and hips squared. Swing arms directly overhead reaching as high as possible, coming on up onto your toes, with full extension in ankles, knees, spine, and shoulders. Once you have reached this extended position, swing your extended arms downward as powerfully as possible, keeping your head neutral or looking forward slightly. Bend more at the hips than knees to initiate greater hamstring tension.

Once you have reached optimal glute and hamstring tension on the downswing, rapidly reverse direction and swing your arms outward and upward. Powerfully extend your hips, knees, and ankles driving the body upward into the air with arms reaching upward as high as possible. Land on two feet with optimal landing mechanics.

Keys to Movement:

1. Stand with feet roughly hip width apart.
2. Perform powerful counter swing movement.
3. Once you have reached optimal hamstring tension on the down swing, swing your warms outward and upward while extending at hips, knees, and ankles.
4. Jump as high as you can.

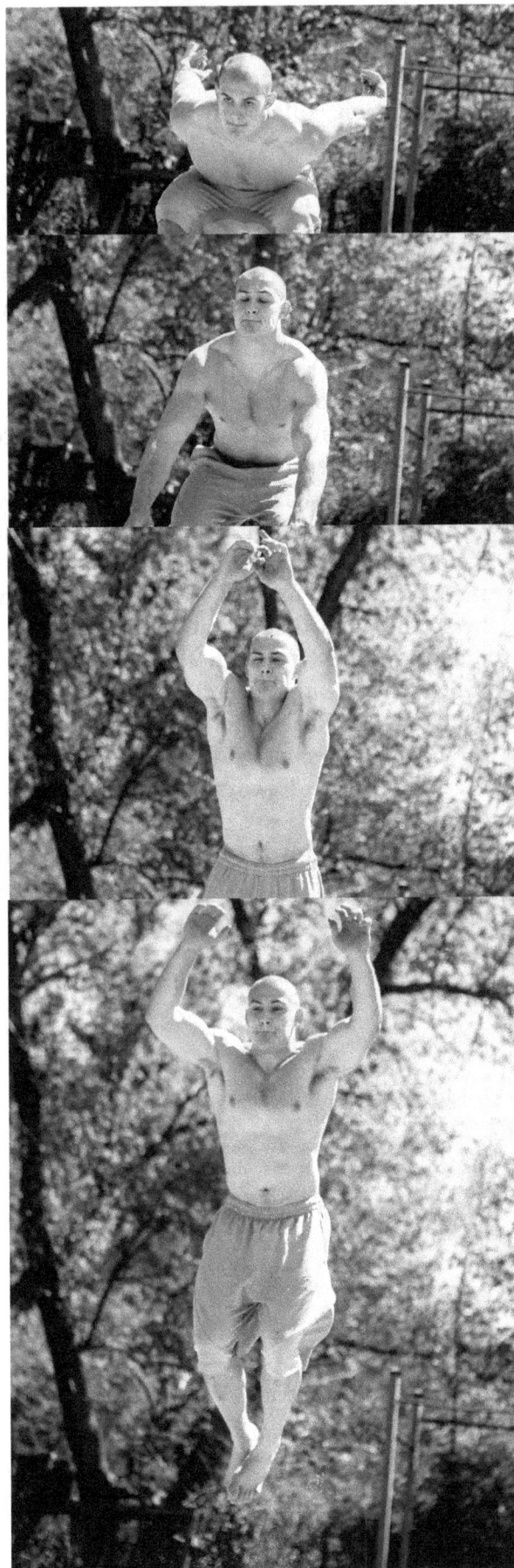

Vertical Jump To Sprint in the Sand

Classification: Total Body Power and Speed

Exercise Prerequisites: Avoid if chronic neck, knee, shoulder or low back pain.

Movement: Perform vertical jump. Upon landing immediately sprint predetermined distance.

Keys to Movement:

1. Utilize proper vertical jump mechanics.
2. Upon controlled landing, immediately sprint out pre-determined distance.

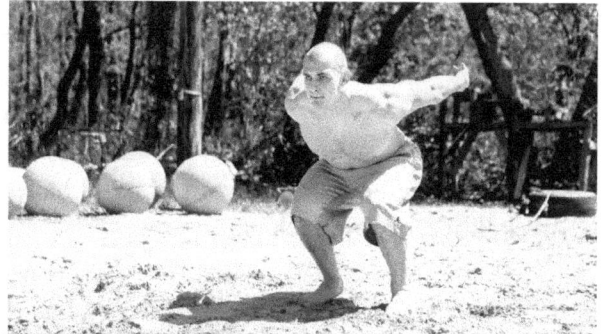

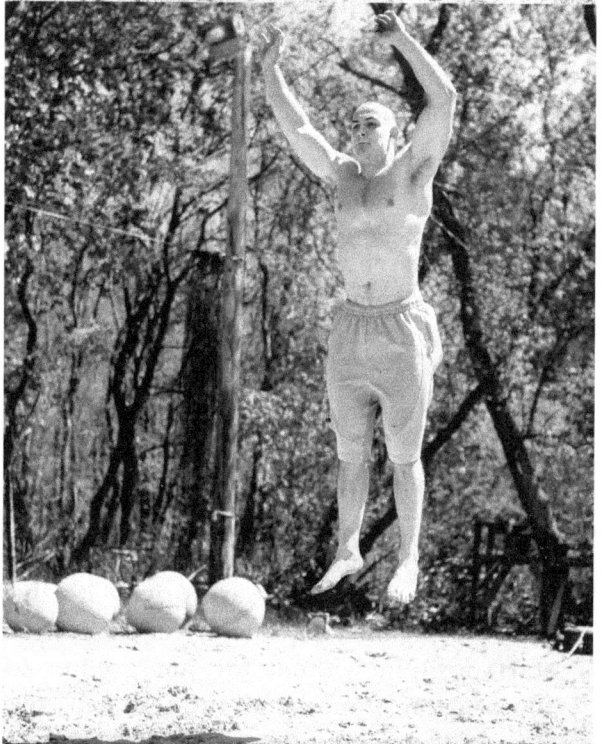

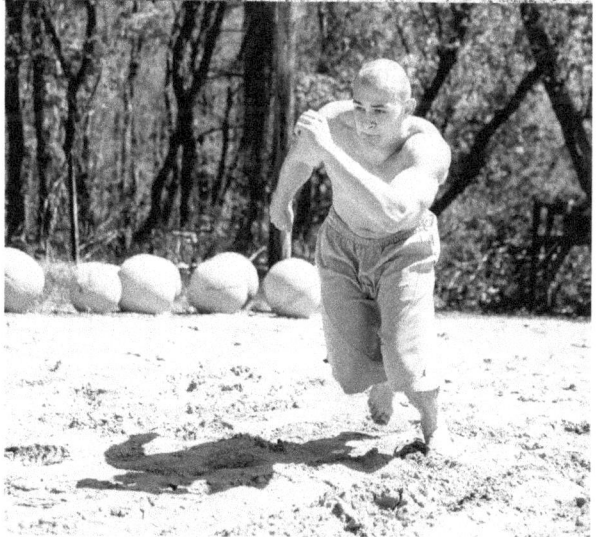

Walking Lunges in the Sand

Classification: Lower Body Strength and Stability

Exercise Prerequisites: Avoid if you have persistent neck, knee, or low back pain.

Movement: Position body with feet hip width apart, torso in neutral/slightly lordotic posture, with dumbbells held at your sides or barbell across the shoulders or in font squat rack position. Maintain upright posture throughout movement. With toes pointing straight ahead, take a large step forward. Lower the hips forward and toward the ground maintaining upright posture with no lean forward. Keeping the back leg as straight as possible, descend until the hamstring comes in contact with the calf on the front leg. It is imperative not to lean forward or allow the front foot heel to come off the ground throughout the movement. As the hamstring comes in the contact with the calf, the knee may cross the toe plane. If the knees are healthy, this can help to strengthen the knee as there is a greater VMO, adductor, hamstring, and gluteal activation with deeper squats and lunges. Once the back knee is 1-2" above the ground initiate the upward/forward drive with the front foot heel, pulling the body forward and up into the original start position without the non-ground contact foot touching the ground until the next step. Keep the torso upright throughout the entire movement. Perform the same for the other leg, driving the knee and lunging forward, performing in a cyclic walking pattern.

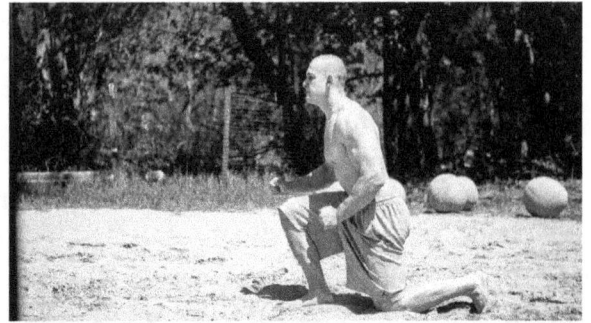

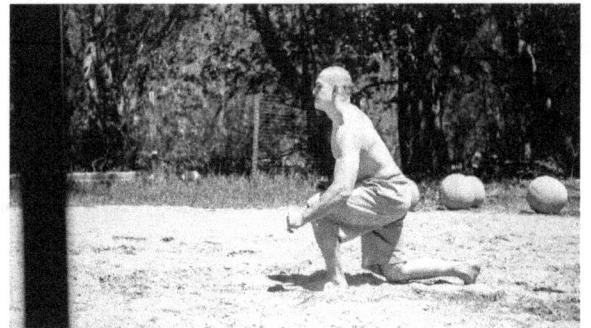

Wheelbarrow Load and Backward Walk

Classification: Total Body Functional Strength and Conditioning

Exercise Prerequisites: Avoid if chronic neck, knee, shoulder or low back pain.

Movement: Position a wheelbarrow next to a small pile of sand. With a short handled shovel load the wheelbarrow as quickly as possible. Feel free to alternate which side you shovel with to avoid development of muscular imbalances. Once you have loaded the wheelbarrow pull it a predetermined distance backward. Dump and perform again.

Keys to Movement:

1. Be sure to alternate shoveling sides to avoid development of muscular imbalances.

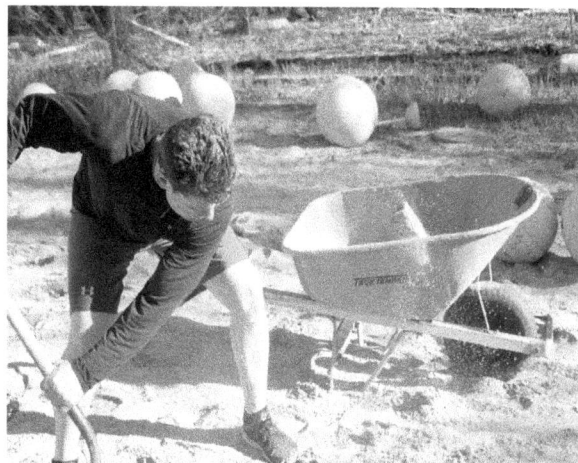

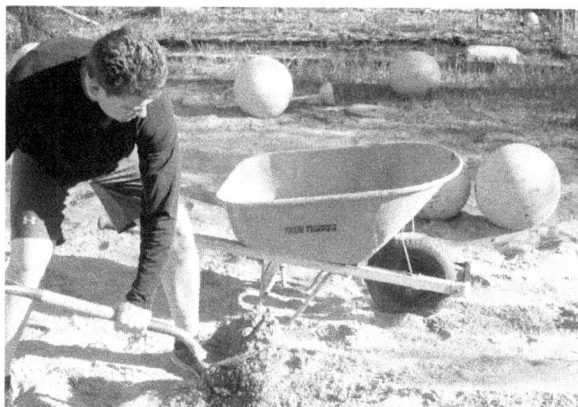

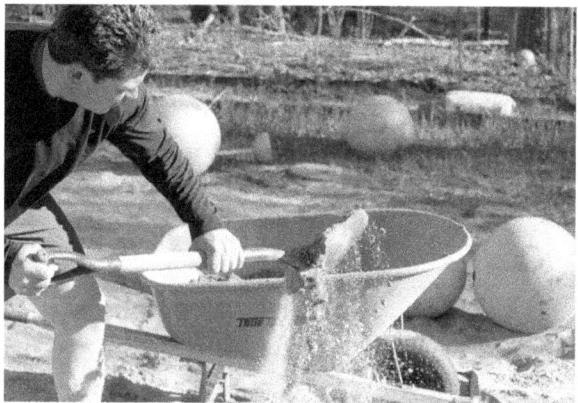

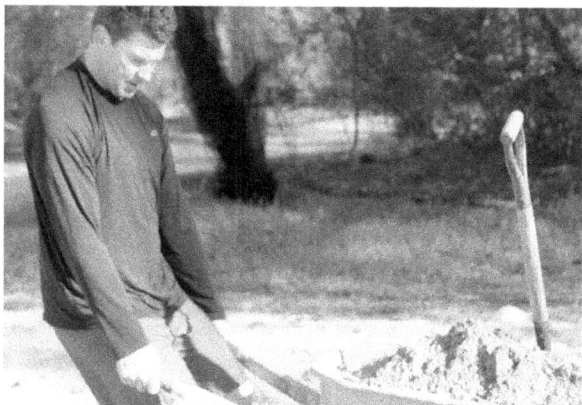

Wheelbarrow Load and Forward Walk

Classification: Total Body Functional Strength and Conditioning

Exercise Prerequisites: Avoid if chronic neck, knee, shoulder or low back pain.

Movement: Position a wheelbarrow next to a small pile of sand. With a short handled shovel load the wheelbarrow as quickly as possible. Feel free to alternate which side you shovel with to avoid development of muscular imbalances. Once you have loaded the wheelbarrow drive it a predetermined distance forward. Dump and perform again.

Keys to Movement:

1. Be sure to alternate shoveling sides to avoid development of muscular imbalances.

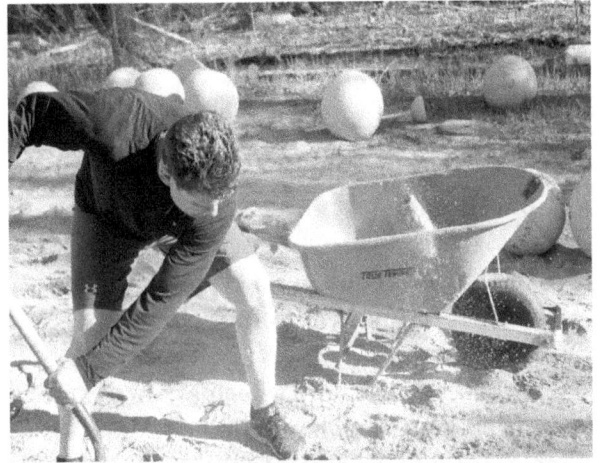

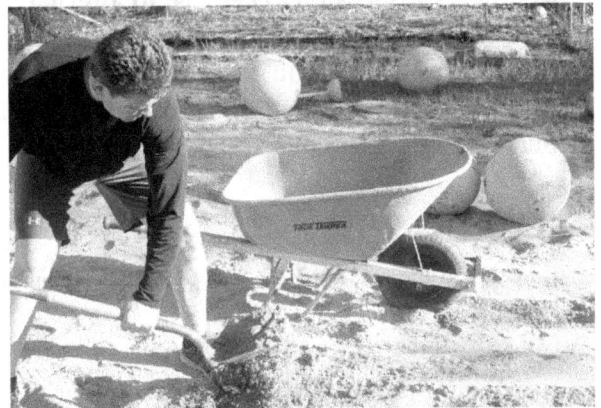

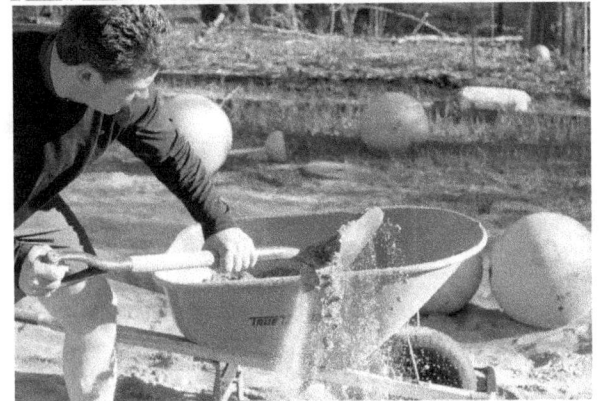

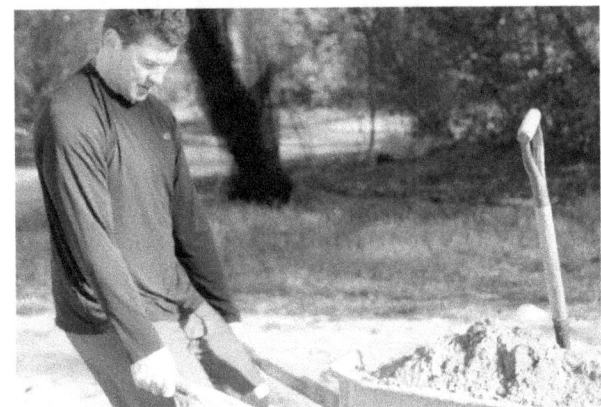

References

1. Anderson A, Meador K, McClure L, Makrozahopoulos D, Brooks D, Mirka G. **A biomechanical analysis of anterior load carriage.** Ergonomics. 50(12); Pp 2104-2117. 2007

2. Bakalar N. **Quicksand Science: Why it traps, how to escape.** *National Geographic News.* 2005.

3. Binnie M, Dawson B, Pinnington H, Landers G, Peeling P. **Sand training: a review of current research and practical applications.** *Journal of Sports Sciences.* 31(1); Pp 8-15. 2014.

4. Binnie M, Dawson B, Arnot M, Pinnington H, Landers G, Peeling P. **Effect of sand versus grass training surfaces during an 8-week pre-season conditioning programme in team sport athletes.** *Journal of Sports Sciences.* 2014.

5. Binnie M, Peeling P, Pinnington H, Landers G, Dawson B. **Effect of surface-specific training on 20-M sprint performance on sand and grass surfaces.** *Journal of Strength and Conditioning Research.* 27(12); Pp 3515-3520. 2013.

6. Binnie M, Dawson B, Pinnington H, Landers G, Peeling P. **Effect of training surface on acute physiological responses after interval training.** *Journal of Strength and Conditioning Research.* 27(4); Pp 1047-1056. 2013.

7. Binnie M, Dawson B, Pinnington H, Landers G, Peeling P. **Part 2: Effect of training surface on acute physiological responses after sport-specific training.** *Journal of Strength and Conditioning Research.* 27(4); Pp 1057-1066. 2013.

8. Bishop D. **A comparison between land and sand-based tests for beach volleyball assessment.** *Journal of Sports Medicine and Physical Fitness.* 43(4); Pp 418-423. 2003.

9. Bryanton M, Kennedy M, Carey J, Chiu L. **Effect of squat depth and barbell load on relative muscular effort in squatting.** *Journal of Strength and Conditioning Research.* 26(10); Pp 2820-2828. 2012.

10. Caterisano A, Moss R, Pellinger T, Woodruff K, Lewis V, Booth W, Khadra T. **The effect of back squat depth on the EMG activity of 4 superficial hip and thigh muscles.** Journal of Strength and conditioning Research. 16(3); Pp 428-432. 2002.

11. Chandler T, Wilson G, Stone M. **The effect of the squat exercise on knee stability.** *Medicine and Science in Sports and Exercise.* 21(3). Pp 299-303. 1989.

12. Crowe J. **Going against the grains.** *The Los Angeles Times.* 2006.

13. Esformes J, Cameron N, Bompouras T. **Postactivation potentiation following different modes of exercise.** *Journal of Strength and Conditioning Research.* 24(7); Pp 1911-1916. 2010

14. Fry A, Kraemer W, Stone M, Warren B, Fleck S, Kearney J, Gordon S. **Endocrine responses to overreaching before and after 1 year of weightlifting.** *Canadian Journal of Applied Physiology.* 19(4); Pp 400-410. 1994

15. Gaudino P, Gaudino Cm Alberti G, Minetti A. **Biomechanics and predicted energetics of sprinting on sand: hints for soccer training.** *Journal of Science and Sports Medicine.* 16(3); Pp 271-275. 2013.

16. Gortsila E, Apostolos T, Nesic G, Maridaki M. **Effect of training surface on agility and passing skills of prepubescent female volleyball players.** *Sports Medicine and Doping Studies.* 3(2); Pp 1-5. 2013.

17. Hakkinen K, Pakarinen A, Alen M, Kauhanen H, Komi P. **Neuromuscular and hormonal responses in elite athletes to two successive strength training sessions in one day.** *European Journal of Applied Physiology and Occupational Physiology.* 57(2); Pp 133-139. 1988

18. Hakkinen K, Pakarinen A, Alen M, Kauhanen H, Komi P. **Daily hormonal and neuromuscular responses to intensive strength training in 1 week.** *International Journal of Sports Medicine.* 9(6); Pp 422-428. 1988.

19. Hall C, Figueroa A, Fernhall B, Kaneley J. **Energy expenditure of walking and running: comparison with prediction equations.** *Medicine and Science in Sports and Exercise.* 36(12); Pp 2128-2134. 2004.

20. Hamlyn N, Behm D, Young W. **Trunk muscle activation during dynamic weight-training exercises and isometric instability activities.** *Journal of Strength and Conditioning Research.* 21(4); Pp 1108-1112. 2007

21. Hartmann H, Wirth K, Klusemann M. **Analysis of the load on the knee joint and vertebral column with changes in depth and weight load.** *Journal of Sports Medicine.* 43; Pp 993-1008. 2013

22. Hartmann H, Wirth K, Klusemann M, Dalic J, Matuschek C, Schmidtbleicher D. **Influence of squatting depth on jumping performance.** *The Journal of Strength and Conditioning Research.* 26(12); Pp 3243-3261. 2012.

23. Hori N, Newton R, Andrews W, Kawamori N, McGuigan M, Nosaka K. **Does performance of hang power clean differentiate performance of jumping, sprinting, and changing of direction?** *Journal of Strength and Conditioning Research.* 22(2); Pp 412-418. 2008.

24. Impellizzeri F, Rampinini E, Castagna C, Martino F, Fiorini S, Wisloff U. **Effect of plyometric training on sand versus grass on muscle soreness and jumping and sprinting ability in soccer players.** *Journal of Sports Medicine.* 42; Pp 42-46. 2008.

25. Johannsen H, Lind T, Jakobsen B, Kroner K. **Exercise-induced knee joint laxity in distance runners.** *British Journal of Sports Medicine.* 23(3); Pp 165-168. 1989

26. Klein K. **The deep squat exercise as utilized in weight training for athletes and its effects on the ligaments of the knee.** *J Assoc Phys Ment Rehabil.* 15; Pp 6-11. 1961

27. Lejeune T, Willems A, Heglund C. **Mechanics and energetics of human locomotion on sand.** *The Journal of Experimental Biology.* 201; Pp 2071-2080. 1998.

28. Mcbride J, Nimphius S, Erickson T. **The acute effects of heavy-load squats and loaded countermovement jumps on sprint performance.** *The Journal of Strength and Conditioning Research.* 19(4); Pp 893-897. 2005.

29. McGill S, McDermott A, Fenwick C. **Comparison of different strongman events: trunk muscle activation and lumbar spine motion, load, and stiffness.** *Journal of Strength and Conditioning Research.* 23(4); Pp 1148-1161. 2009

30. Meyers E. **Effect of selected exercise variables on ligament stability and flexibility of the knee.** *Research Quarterly.* 42(4); Pp 411-422. 1971.

31. Miyama M, Nosaka K. **Influence of surface on muscle damage and soreness induced by consecutive drop jumps**. *Journal of Strength and Conditioning Research.* 18(2); Pp 206-211. 2004

32. Mujika I, Santisteban J, Castagna C. **In-season effect of short term sprint and power training programs on elite junior soccer players.** *Journal of Strength and Conditioning Research.* 23(9); Pp 2581-2587. 2009.

33. Oviatt R, Hemba G. **Oregon State: Sandblasting through the PAC.** *National Strength and Conditioning Association Journal.* 13(4); 1991. Pp 40-46.

34. Panariello R, Backus S, Parker J. **The effect of the squat exercise on anterior-posterior knee translation in professional football players.** *American Journal of Sports Medicine.* 22(6); Pp 768-773. 1994

35. Riggs M, Sheppard J. **The relative importance of strength and power qualities to vertical jump height of elite beach volleyball players during the countermovement and squat jump.** *The Journal of Human Sport and Exercise Online.* 4(4); Pp 221-236. 2009.

36. Shea J. Lean Body Solutions. APECS Publishing LLC. 2012.

37. Shea J. The In-Season Training Manual. APECS Publishing LLC. 2012.

38. Siff, M. *Supertraining.* Denver, Co. Pp 268. 2003.

39. Steiner M, Grana W, Chilag K, Schelberg-Karnes E. **The effect of exercise on anterior-posterior knee laxity.** *American Journal of Sports Medicine.* 14(1); Pp 24-29. 1986

40. Stone M, Sands W, Pierce K, Carlock J, Cardinale M, Newton R. **Relationship of maximum strength to weightlifting performance.** *Medicine and Science In Sports and Exercise.* 37(6); Pp 1037-1043. 2005.

41. Tricoli V, Lamas L, Carnevale R, Ugrinowitsch C. **Short-term effects on lower-body functional power development: weightlifting vs. vertical jump training programs.** *Journal of Strength and Conditioning Research.* 19(2); Pp 433-437. 2005.

42. Zimmerman P. **He can run, but he can't hide.** *Sports Illustrated.* 1982.

About The Author

With over 16 years of practical experience as a coach and educator, Jason Shea has earned a reputation as a strength coach and body composition specialist capable of training athletes and trainees at the highest levels. As the owner of APECS (www.apec-s.com) and CrossFit Tri-Valley (www.crossfit-trivalley.com) Jason has earned the distinguished honor of being recognized as one of less than a dozen PICP Level IV International Strength Coaches in the U.S. His clientele has included professional, college, high school, and Olympic hopeful athletes as well as Fortune 500 business executives, SWAT Teams, military personnel, state and local firefighters, and more than 40 local high school, club, and college teams.

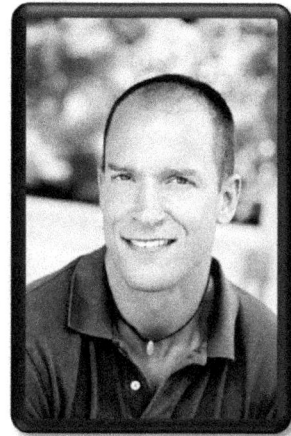

He has been strength coach to 2 High School Super Bowl Teams, 5 State Champion Lacrosse Teams, numerous State and New England Champion wrestlers and track athletes, Boston Globe Players of the year in Football, Volleyball, Wrestling, Lacrosse, and Soccer, over 25 High School and College league MVP's from all sports, College and high school league all-stars in nearly every sport, and league champion teams in high school sports including Football, Field Hockey, Soccer, Basketball, Hockey, Baseball, Field Hockey, Lacrosse, Wrestling, and Softball.

Jason holds a Bachelor's Degree in Exercise Science and a Master's in Human Movement. He has been certified through various organizations including the USAW, NASM, NSCA, ISSA, ACE, and PICP. Not one to rest on his laurels, Jason has traveled throughout the US and Europe to learn the most effective techniques in training, soft tissue, nutrition, and body composition taught by the Poliquin Strength Institute and PICP Certification Program.

Along with his role as Head Strength Coach at APECS and CrossFit Tri-Valley Jason is also the Massachusetts Statewide Health and Wellness Coordinator for the Municipal Police Training Committee. In this role he is responsible for academy certification and dissemination of continuing education for municipal police officers teaching at the Municipal Police Academies in Massachusetts.

The success of his business and clientele has led to current positions as Adjunct Professor in the Sport Fitness department at Dean College, consulting Strength Coach to the highly successful Dean College Football and Soccer Teams, Performance Director for the Speed and Power Academy at Franklin High School, Strength and Conditioning Coach to the nationally ranked Boston Irish Wolfhounds Rugby Team, columnist for the Metrowest Daily News, and the opportunity to co-author Law Enforcement articles with world renowned strength coach Charles Poliquin. He has also been a featured lecturer on strength and conditioning topics for various organizations including local colleges, corporation and high schools, Blue Chip Football Camps, and club teams in all sports.

Most important to Jason is the time he spends with his inspirations; son Ayden, daughter Bryn, and beautiful wife Wendy.

www.ingramcontent.com/pod-product-compliance
Lightning Source LLC
Chambersburg PA
CBHW081647270326
41933CB00018B/3374